T0074357

This book has been sponsored by Ethicon Endo-Surgery (Europe) GmbH and Johnson & Johnson MEDICAL GmbH, Norderstedt, Germany. The author is responsible for the content of the publication. Information provided in this book is offered in good faith as an educational tool for health care professionals. The information has been thoroughly reviewed and is believed to be useful and accurate at the time of its publication, but is offered without warranty of any kind. The author and the sponsors shall not be responsible for any loss or damage arising from its use.

OPERATION PRIMER **volume 8**

Laparoscopic Gastric Banding

Editors

Marc Immenroth
Jürgen Brenner

Author

Karl Miller

assisted by

Birgit Wahl

Maike Aukstinnis
Ann-Katrin Güler
Astrid Künemund
Annegret Röhling
Detlev Ruge
Sabine Schroeder

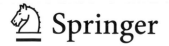

Author

Karl Miller, M.D., FACS
Associate Professor of Surgery, Head of the Surgical Department, Krankenhaus Hallein,
Bürgermeisterstr. 34,
5400 Hallein, Austria

Editors

Marc Immenroth, PhD
Senior Marketing Manager EP Austria & Plus Platform & Synthetic Absorbables D-A-CH,
Johnson & Johnson MEDICAL GmbH,
Robert-Koch-Straße 1,
22851 Norderstedt, Germany

Jürgen Brenner, M.D.
Director European Surgical Institute,
Johnson & Johnson MEDICAL GmbH,
Hummelsbütteler Steindamm 71,
22851 Norderstedt, Germany

ISBN 978-3-642-19274-6 Laparoscopic Gastric Banding

Bibliografische Information der Deutschen Bibliothek
The Deutsche Bibliothek lists this publication in Deutsche Nationalbibliografie;
detailed bibliographic data are available in the internet at http://dnb.ddb.de.

First published in Germany in 2011 by Springer Medizin Verlag
springer.com

© Ethicon Endo-Surgery (Europe) GmbH

SPIN 80035214
Layout and typesetting: Dr. Carl GmbH, Stuttgart, Germany
Printing: Stürtz GmbH, Würzburg, Germany

18/5135/DK – 5 4 3 2 1 0

EDITORS' PREFACE

This Operation Primer marks the continuation of a series of very successful books, which have gained ever more recognition in recent years. Thanks to consistently positive reviews in renowned specialist publications in both England and Germany, we are motivated to continue to invest in these 'cook books' for surgeons. In response to international demand we plan to release the forthcoming English-language primers in other languages. In addition to the central European languages, Chinese will also be available.

The idea for the Operation Primer series originated in a scientific study entitled "Mental Training in Surgical Education" that formed part of a collaborative project between the surgical department of the University of Cologne, the Institute of Sports and Sports Science of the University of Heidelberg and the European Surgical Institute (ESI) in Norderstedt. The aim of the study was to evaluate the effect of mental training, which has been used successfully in top-class sports for decades, on surgical training. However, in order for mental training to be applied to surgery, it first had to undergo modification. In the course of this modification, the first Operation Primer was produced, the layout of which was largely adopted for the final version presented here.

The practice of defining nodal points for operations and then learning these by heart and going through them mentally has been proven to lead to better surgical results. Surgeons approach operations more prepared, are no longer surprised when confronted with the unexpected, and thus operate with more confidence.

This latest primer focuses on a current topic: surgery for morbid obesity. Gastric banding is one of the techniques that has proven useful, in the hands of experts and when performed at the right time.

Our next primers on the topic of bariatric surgery will offer further techniques, broken down into and presented as nodal points. This further proves the value of the nodal point philosophy for greater patient safety. Each operation will be presented in a book which concentrates on the essentials. There are suggestions of potential dangers and their avoidance, presentation of technical procedures and consideration of anatomical variety. Furthermore, the formulation of an operation note will help to improve the quality of documentation.

An expert in the field of bariatrics, *Karl Miller,* has worked to develop this Operation Primer in accordance with the mental training methods which are a staple of previous editions. Each nodal point has been carefully and collaboratively defined and is aligned with the most sensible course of action; these points should be consecutively observed.

We have also received excellent support from *Dr. Carl GmbH*, which has accompanied us at each stage of the working process and has contributed greatly to making these innovative surgical textbooks what they are. The diagrams, line drawings, etc. were produced mainly by *Thomas Heller. Detlev Ruge* was responsible for the pictures featured in this Operation Primer. The existing concept of practical surgical primers has become reality through the publishing company *Springer Medizin Verlag Heidelberg.* Sincere thanks to all of them.

Above all else, patient safety is our main aim, and we hope that our books will assist the reader in achieving this goal.

The Editors   March 2011

"It is difficult to make it simple" – I think about this quotation from Pablo Picasso every day in surgery. It is a matter of summarizing complex working steps and treatments "simply". Obesity surgery is not only a craft; it also signifies consideration of the disease as a whole. This Operation Primer undertakes the task of communicating basic surgical techniques. Only someone who knows all the technical possibilities and procedures is in a position to react flexibly and adequately in different situations.

About 50 different surgical methods have been developed in obesity surgery in the past 50 years. It is obvious from this that the optimal surgical method for the obese patient does not exist. Among the stomach-narrowing surgical methods, the adjustable gastric band has become established as a very effective and minimally invasive surgical procedure. Experience has shown that peri- and postoperative complications can be reduced with different band placements and also with simplified working steps. This Operation Primer is an ideal format for communicating new operative methods, but it does not replace training by an experienced surgeon.

A surgeon cannot rest on his laurels but must always keep up with the latest techniques. I would therefore like to take this opportunity to thank the European Surgical Institute (ESI) for making mental training, training on the computer simulator and operations in the laboratory possible. First-class surgery is possible only through careful acquisition of knowledge, regular training and quality control.

Karl Miller   March 2011

AUTHOR

Karl Miller, M.D., FACS

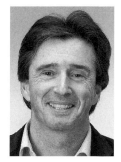

– Studied Medicine in Innsbruck, Austria
– 1983 Doctorate in Medicine at the University of Innsbruck, Austria
– 1991 Qualified as General Surgeon
– 1995–2000 Vice Chief at the 2nd Surgical Department of the General Hospital Salzburg, Austria
– 1996 Associate Professor of Surgery at the University of Innsbruck, Austria
– Since 1996 Faculty of the European Surgical Institute (ESI) in Norderstedt, Germany
– Since 2001 Head of the Surgical Department of the Hospital Hallein, Austria
– Since 2003 Associate Editor of the Journal *Obesity Surgery*
– Since 2008 Associate Editor of the *European Journal of Obesity*

Focus of Research and Work
– Bariatric Surgery
– Surgical Education

Experience
– Developed and standardized the surgical technique for laparoscopic gastric banding (pars flaccida technique)
– Experienced in laparoscopic gastric surgery and laparoscopic functional surgery of the stomach (Nissen and Toupet fundoplicatio)
– 1999 Organized the World Congress on Obesity Surgery in Salzburg, Austria
– Since 2003 has organized 20 international workshops per year where more than 650 surgeons worldwide were given "hands-on" training in laparoscopic gastric banding and gastric bypass

Author of many scientific articles in surgical journals

Contents

Appendices

Introduction

From an educational point of view, the Operation Primer is somewhat plagiaristic. The layout – and this can be admitted freely – is largely taken over from commonly available cook books. In such books, the ingredients and cooking utensils required to prepare the recipe in question are normally listed first. The most important cooking procedures are then described briefly in the text. Photographs support the written explanations and show what the dish should look like when prepared. Sometimes diagrams and illustrations make individual cooking steps clearer.

Despite these obvious parallels, there is a crucial difference between cook books and the Operation Primer: in the Operation Primer, complicated and complex surgical techniques are described that are intended to help the surgeon and his team perform an operation safely and economically. Ultimately, it always comes down to the patient's welfare. The following must therefore be said early in this introduction:

- The use of the Operation Primer as an aid to operating requires that surgical techniques have first been completely mastered.

- Being alert to possible mistakes is categorically the most important principle when operating; avoiding mistakes is crucial.

As already mentioned in the Editors' preface, the concept of the Operation Primer originated in a scientific study with the title "Mental Training in Surgical Education" that formed part of a collaborative project between the surgical department of the University of Cologne (under Prof. Hans Troidl), the Institute of Sports and Sports Science of the University of Heidelberg, and the European Surgical Institute (ESI) in Norderstedt. Laparoscopic cholecystectomy was the initial focus.

Mental training is derived from top-class sports. This is understood as methodically repeating and consciously imagining actions and movements without actually carrying them out at the same time (cf. Driskell, Copper & Moran, 1994; Feltz & Landers, 1983; Immenroth, 2003; Immenroth, Eberspächer & Hermann, 2008). Scientific involvement with imagining movement has a long tradition in medical and psychological research. As early as 1852, Lotze described how imagining and perceiving movements can lead to a concurrent performance "with quiet movements …" (Lotze, 1852). This phenomenon later became known by the names "Ideomotion" and "Carpenter effect" (Carpenter, 1874).

In the collaborative project, mental training was modified in such a way that it could be employed in the training and further education of young surgeons. In mental training in surgery, surgeons visualize the operation from the inner perspective without performing any actual movements, i.e., they go through the operation step by step in their mind's eye. In the study that was conducted at the ESI, the first Operation Primer was used as the basis for this visualization. In this primer, laparoscopic cholecystectomy was subdivided into individual, clearly depicted steps, the so-called nodal points.

The study evaluated the effect of the mental training on learning laparoscopic cholecystectomy compared with practical training and with a control group. The planning, conduct, and evaluation of the study took seven years (2000–2007), with over 100 surgeons participating.

The results corresponded exactly with the expectations: the mentally trained surgeons improved in a similar degree to those surgeons who received additional practical training on a pelvi trainer simulator (in some subscales even more). Moreover, there was greater improvement in these two groups compared with the control group, which did not receive any additional mental or practical training (cf. in detail, Immenroth, Bürger, Brenner, Nagelschmidt, Eberspächer & Troidl, 2007; Immenroth, Bürger, Brenner, Kemmler, Nagelschmidt, Eberspächer & Troidl, 2005; Immenroth, Eberspächer, Nagelschmidt, Troidl, Bürger, Brenner, Berg, Müller & Kemmler, 2005).

Recently, a significant improvement in surgical knowledge and confidence was shown by both experienced and novice surgeons in another study about mental training in laparoscopic surgery (Arora et al., 2010). Therefore, mental training can be seen as a cost- and time-effective training tool that should be integrated into surgical training.

Furthermore, the study of Immenroth et al. (2007) included a questionnaire to determine the extent to which the mentally trained surgeons accepted mental training as a teaching method in surgery. Mental training was assessed as very positive by all 34 mentally trained surgeons. The Operation Primer received particular acclaim in the evaluation:

- 82 % of the surgeons wished to use similar self-made Operation Primers in their daily work.

- 85 % of the surgeons attributed the success of the mental training at least in part to the Operation Primer.

- 88 % of the surgeons wanted to have these Operation Primers as a fixed component of the course at the ESI.

This positive response to the study was the starting point for the production of the present series of Operation Primers.

Prior to publication, the Operation Primer was developed by methodical and didactical means and then adapted to the readers' needs and wishes. This was carried out following a survey of 93 surgeons (interns, resident doctors, assistant medical directors and medical directors) who participated in surgical courses at the ESI. They evaluated in detail the structure and components by means of a questionnaire.

The results of this survey gave important findings on how to optimize the Operation Primer. The sense and representation of the nodal points, the comprehensibility and detail of the text, and the photographs of the operation were highly valued especially by young surgeons (Güler, Immenroth, Berg, Bürger & Gawad, 2006). The comprehensive research undertaken with this Operation Primer series will ensure its overall value to the reader.

Structure and handling of the Operation Primer

In the present series of Operation Primers, an attempt has been made to standardize the described laparoscopic operations as much as possible. This is achieved first by applying the same format to all operating techniques described. Second, operative sequences that are performed identically in all operations are always explained using the same blocks of text. By following a general structure for the description of all operations and by using identical text blocks, it was intended to aid recognition of recurring patterns and their translation into action even for different operations.

The Operation Primer is divided into five chapters, each identified by Roman numerals and different register colors on the margin. The contents of the individual chapters will now be explained.

In **Preparations for the operation,** the basic instruments for all laparoscopic operations and then the additional instruments for the specific operation are listed. This is followed by a detailed description of the preparing of the gastric band, the positioning and shaving of the patient, attaching the neutral electrode, setting up the equipment, skin disinfection and sterile draping of the patient. The operative preparation is concluded with a detailed description and an illustration of how the operating team is to be positioned for the operation in question.

In the chapter **Creating the pneumoperitoneum – placing the trocar for the scope,** three alternatives are shown in detail: the Hasson method, trocar with optical obturator, and Veress needle. The choice of method is up to the individual surgeon. All three alternatives are employed in surgical practice. However, it should be pointed out that the greatest danger in minimally invasive surgery is the insertion of the Veress needle, as it is done "blind".

Placing the working trocars is explained in detail in the next chapter. The written explanations are supplemented by a diagram. In order to keep a constant overview of the placement of the trocars, even during the following description of the operation sequence, this illustration is shown in diminished size in every single operative step.

The core of the Operation Primer is the chapter **Nodal points.** This is where the actual sequence of the operation is described in detail. However, prior to this detailed explanation, the term nodal point will be explained briefly. In the Editors' preface and introduction, mental training was mentioned as a form of training used successfully in top-class sports for decades, and this is where the term originates. In sports as in surgery, a nodal point is understood as one of those structural components of movement that are absolutely essential for performing the movement optimally. Nodal points have to be passed through in succession and are characterized by a reduction in the degrees of freedom of action. In mental training they act as orientation points for methodical repetition and conscious imagining of the athletic or operative movement (cf. in detail Immenroth et al., 2008).

For every operation in the Operation Primer series, these nodal points were extracted in a prolonged process by the authors in collaboration with the editors. The nodal points represent the basic structural framework of an operation. Because of their particular relevance and for better orientation, all of the nodal points in the Operation Primer are shown on the left on each double page as a flow chart. The current nodal point is highlighted graphically. The instruments required for this nodal point and the specific trocars for it are listed in a box on the right, beside the flow chart.

Below the instrument box, instructions regarding the nodal point are given as briefly as possible. According to Miller (1956), people can best store 7±2 units of information ("Magical number 7"). Therefore, no more than seven single instructions are listed per nodal point, if possible. With re-

I	Preparations for the operation
II	Creating the pneumoperitoneum – placing the trocar for the scope
III	Placing the working trocars
IV	Nodal points
V	Management of difficult situations and complications
	Appendices

3 possibilities for creating the pneumoperitoneum: the choice is up to the surgeon

Veress needle = greatest danger!

Continuous illustration of the trocar positions

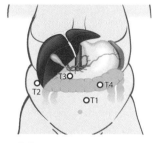

Nodal point = term from top-class sports

Nodal points:
1) absolutely essential
2) successive order
3) no degrees of freedom

Flow chart of the sequence of nodal points on each double page

Maximum of 7±2 instructions per nodal point

gard to the instructions, it should be noted that the change of instruments between the individual nodal points is not described explicitly as a rule; rather, this is apparent through different instruments in the instrument box.

Where necessary, particular moments where special attention is needed are pointed out in red.

Watch outs are pointed out in red!

The described operation sequence is only one way of performing the operation safely and economically, namely the way preferred by the authors. Undoubtedly, a number of other equally valid operation sequences exist. As far as possible, notes on alternative methods are given in small blue print at the end of each nodal point.

Alternatives: In small blue print at the end of the nodal point.

In the fifth chapter, the **Management of difficult situations and complications** is described in detail. In general, details on adhesions, bleeding, injuries to organs, etc. are given first.

Illustration of anatomical variations, an example of an operation note and details about postoperative management, band adjustment and postoperative complications in the appendices

In the **Appendices** relevant anatomical variations which can occur in the operation sequence and may require a different approach are described first. In order to give the Operation Primer even more practical relevance, an example of an operation note is then reproduced. The appendices also contain helpful hints for the postoperative management, detailed information about band adjustment and about postoperative complications and their management, as well as the bibliographical references and list of keywords.

In order to avoid repetition, reference is made throughout the text to relevant chapters of the Operation Primer, if necessary. To do this, the Roman numeral of the chapter and the number of the corresponding section are shown in parentheses. Referral is made most often to the fifth chapter, where the management of difficult situations and complications is described. These references are set off in red letters.

(→ p. 66, V-4) = reference to the 4th section of chapter V

All sources in the literature are listed in the bibliography

Finally, it must be pointed out that for better readability of the Operation Primer no bibliographical references at all are given in the text. However, in order to give an overview of the basic and more extensive sources, the entire literature is listed in the bibliography.

Make sure that the following preoperative requirements for laparoscopic gastric banding have been met:

- The indication for the operation is correct.
- The patient has given detailed informed written consent.
- The bowel is prepared appropriately prior to laparoscopic gastrointestinal surgery.
- Thromboprophylaxis (low-molecular-weight heparin) has been given as per local practice.
- Single-dose perioperative antibiotic prophylaxis has been given.

Basic instruments

- Size 11 scalpel
- 10-ml syringe with 0.9 % NaCl solution
- Dissecting scissors
- 2 Langenbeck hooks
- Suction device
- Needle holder
- Suture scissors
- 2 surgical forceps
- 2 Backhaus clamps
- Compresses
- Swabs with an integral X-ray contrast strip
- Sutures:
    - Fascia: 2–0 absorbable, polyfilament
    - Subcutaneous: 3–0 absorbable, polyfilament, if necessary
    - Skin: 4–0 or 5–0 absorbable, monofilament
- Trocar side closure device, if necessary
- Skin adhesive, if necessary
- Dressings

Instruments for the first access, depending on the type of access:
a) Hasson method:
    - Hasson trocar (10/12 mm)
    - 2 retaining sutures (2–0)
    - Purse-string suture (2–0)
b) Trocar with optical obturator (e.g. Endopath XCEL® bladeless trocar, Ethicon Endo-Surgery)
c) Veress needle (e.g. Endopath® Veress Needle Ultra, Ethicon Endo-Surgery)

There should always be a basic laparotomy set in the operating room so that in an emergency a laparotomy can be performed without delay!

Additional instruments for laparoscopic gastric banding

Trocars:	(e.g. Endopath XCEL® trocar, Ethicon Endo-Surgery)
T1: Trocar for the scope	(10/12 mm)
T2: Working trocar	(5 mm or 10/12 mm; depending on the liver retracting device)
T3: Working trocar	(5 mm or 10/12 mm)
T4: Working trocar	(15 mm; for insertion of the gastric band)

- Additional trocars, if necessary
- Reducer caps, if necessary
- Angled scope (0° scope, if necessary, for trocar with optical obturator)

Extra-long trocars are usually not required. The only instrument that should always be extra-long is the HF (high frequency) hook!

- SAGB (Swedish Adjustable Gastric Band) Velocity Curved (Ethicon Endo-Surgery*)

Before using the SAGB Gastric Band read the instructions for use and become familiar with the band! Ensure that an additional gastric band is available in case of damage to the gastric band!

- 10-ml syringe
- Endoscopic Dissection and Gastric Band Retrieval System (e.g. Goldfinger™, Ethicon Endo-Surgery*)
- Injection Port and Applier (e.g. Velocity™, Ethicon Endo-Surgery*)
- 2 Langenbeck hooks
- Huber needle (used to aspirate air from the injection port)
- Liver retracting device with fixation arm
- Additional liver retracting device with fixation arm, if necessary
- Extra-long HF (high frequency) electrode handle and hook
- Curved dissector
- 2 atraumatic grasping forceps (5 mm and/or 10 mm)
- Dissecting swab
- Curved scissors
- Needle holder
- Sutures for safety sutures between diaphragm, fundus and pouch (2–0 non-absorbable, polyfilament)
- Suction-irrigation instrument

For the anesthetist:
- Gastric calibration tube 180° asymmetrical balloon (e.g. Gastric Calibration Tube, Ethicon Endo-Surgery*)
- 30-ml syringe
- 25 ml saline solution, if necessary
- 5 ml methylene blue 1 %
- 15 ml saline solution
- 10-ml syringe with cannula
- Small bowl

Alternatives: Instead of the HF (high frequency) electrode, an ultrasonic device (e.g. Harmonic ACE® shears, Ethicon Endo-Surgery) can be used. To place the safety sutures the Endo-Suture-System® with a knot pusher can be used as an alternative to a needle holder.

* Manufactured by Obtech Medical Sàrl and marketed by Ethicon Endo-Surgery

Basic instruments

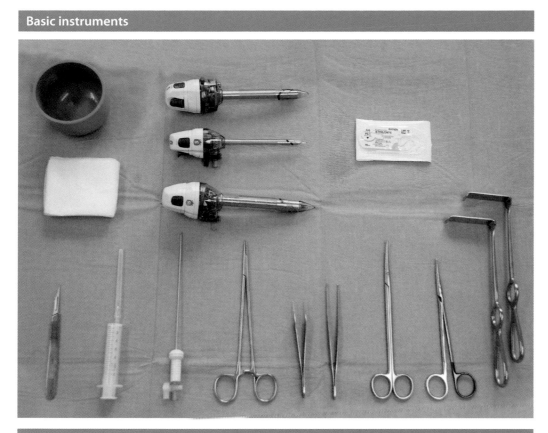

Additional instruments for laparoscopic gastric banding

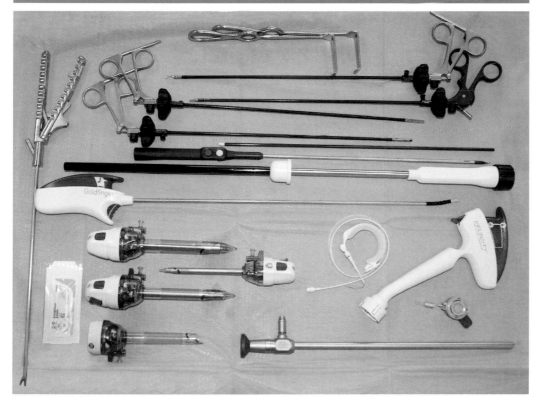

SAGB Gastric Band

1 Reinforcing band
2 Band extender
3 Extender strap including black cutting indicator
4 Extender cutting groove
5 Pre-lock flanges
6 Suture loop
7 Buckle tab
8 Locking shell
9 Unlocking grip
10 Balloon
11 Tubing (catheter)
12 One-way valve
13 Locking connector
14 Velocity™ Injection Port

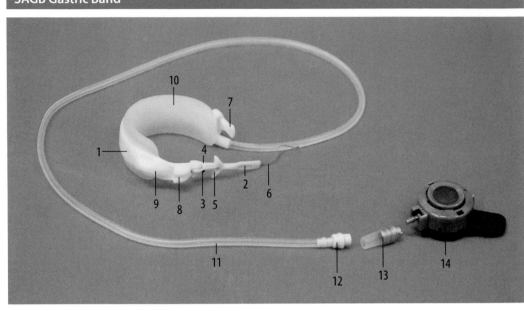

Velocity™ Injection Port and Applier

1 Injection port
2 Port septum
3 Actuator ring including lock/ unlock indicator
4 Locking connector
5 Locking connector tab
6 Connection tube
7 Connection housing
8 Band tubing
9 Tubing strain relief
10 Safety cap
11 Port applier
12 Handle
13 Firing lever
14 Safety release trigger
15 Guide notch
16 Applier shaft
17 Applier receptacle
18 Guide notch indicator
19 Lock/unlock indicator
20 Suture hole
21 SAGB Gastric Band with attached Velocity™ Injection Port
22 Band extender
23 Extender strap including black cutting indicator
24 Buckle tab
25 Buckle tongue including lock indicator

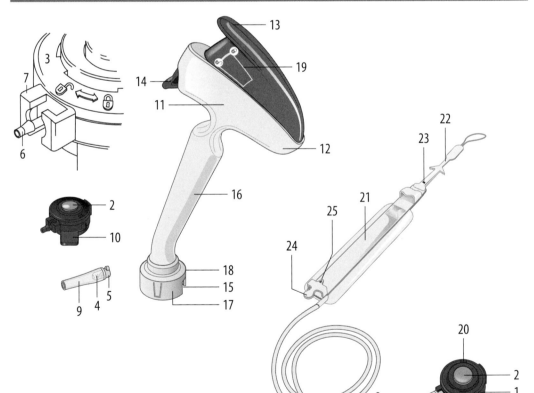

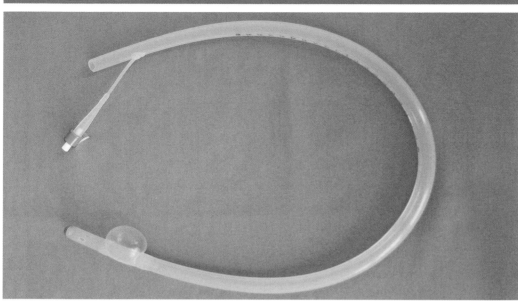

Preparing the gastric band

Make sure that the gastric band, the tubing system and the port are intact and complete!

In order to check the gastric band for leaks, attach a 10-ml syringe filled with 11 ml of air to the one-way valve of the band. Fill the gastric band with 11 ml of air.

Take care not to fill in more than 11 ml of air in order not to damage the balloon.

Then immerse it in a bowl of sterile saline solution and look for air bubbles in the water emanating from the balloon or the tubing. The presence of bubbles indicates a leak in the balloon or tubing.

In case of a leak in the balloon or tubing, use a new SAGB Gastric Band.

Withdraw all air from the balloon with the syringe. It is important that the balloon and the tubing are free of air during the initial placement of the band.

Make sure that the balloon and the tubing are free of air during the initial placement of the band!

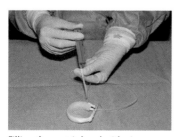
Filling the gastric band with air

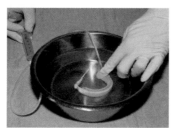
Immersing the gastric band in sterile saline solution

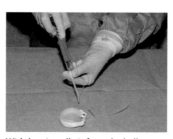
Withdrawing all air from the balloon

Emptying the urinary bladder

- In order to avoid injuries to the urinary bladder, make sure that the patient's bladder is emptied preoperatively by placing a temporary transurethral catheter.

Positioning of the patient

The technical fittings, especially the operating table, must be approved and functional for the patient's weight!

- Position the patient in lithotomy position.

- Stretch thighs and legs apart with a slight flexure.

- Place both arms at an angle not greater than 70° to the long axis of the body in order to avoid injuries to the axillary nerve.

- Pad the shoulder, elbow and knee joints in order to avoid pressure injuries, particularly of the nerves.

- For better positioning of the patient, hyperextend the back in the lumbar region by means of a pad or by appropriate adjustment of the operating table.

- Use a padded board as a surface to lie on to prevent the patient from sliding when put in extreme positions.

- After creating the pneumoperitoneum and inserting the trocar for the scope (→ p. 25, II) and the scope (→ p. 30, III) put the patient in a reverse Trendelenburg position (30°).

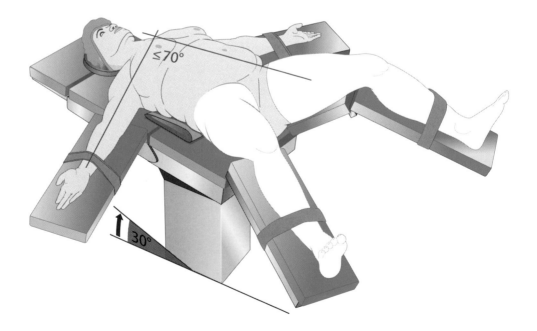

Shaving

- Shave the patient from the mamillae to above the pubic symphysis and from the left to the right anterior superior iliac spine in order to be able to convert to a conventional operation if complications occur.
- If monopolar current is used, shave the adhesion side for the neutral electrode (as close as possible to the operating field, e.g. on the upper thigh).

Neutral electrode

- Before placing the neutral electrode, ensure that the skin at this site and all skin areas in contact with the table are absolutely dry.
- Then stick the entire surface of the electrode carefully above the greatest possible muscle mass (e.g. on the upper thigh). The conducting cable must be at the greatest possible distance from the operating field.

When using monopolar current, always guard against burns on moist areas of the skin due to current!

Setting up the equipment

- Set the generator of the HF electrode to an appropriate power level for the intended use.
- Position the foot pedal.
- Attach the suction-irrigation instrument.
- Select a maximum pressure of 12 mmHg on the CO_2 insufflator (with a flow of 6–8 l/min).

Skin disinfection

- Disinfect the skin from the mamillae to the pubic symphysis. Pay particular attention to careful disinfection of all skin folds.

Sterile draping

- Drape the operating field with sterile drapes so that it is limited cranially at the level of the xiphoid, just above the umbilicus caudally, and by the midaxillary lines laterally.
- While sterile draping of the operating field, position the fixation arm of the liver retracting device at the right side of the table on the level of the liver.

Positioning of the operating team

- The surgeon stands between the patient's spread legs.

- The camera assistant stands to the left at the level of the patient's pelvis.

- The scrub nurse stands to the right at the level of the patient's knee.

- The monitor is located in the line of vision of the surgeon and the camera assistant, hanging behind the patient's head.

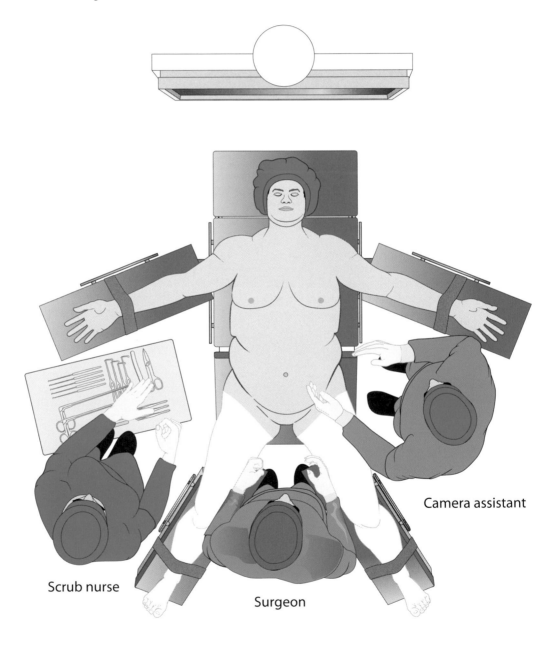

Scrub nurse

Camera assistant

Surgeon

Alternative: If a ceiling monitor is not available, position the monitor in the line of vision of the surgeon and the camera assistant on the right at the level of the patient's head.

Creating the pneumoperitoneum – placing the trocar for the scope

There are three ways of creating a pneumoperitoneum, which will be described in detail below:

a) Hasson method (open technique)

b) Trocar with optical obturator

c) Veress needle (closed technique)

> Because of the large variety of trocars available and the resulting variety of methods of introducing the trocars, follow their individual instruction manuals!

> Note the following special features when creating the pneumoperitoneum in laparoscopic obesity surgery:
> - The thickness of the abdominal wall may require a bigger incision, which may make gas-proof placement of the Hasson trocar difficult (→ p. 26, IIa)!
> - Use of an optical obturator in the trocar has proven to be helpful in obesity surgery (→ p. 27, IIb)!
> - Select the access for the Veress needle in the left upper abdomen in order to minimize the injury risk of patients with hepatomegaly (→ p. 28, IIc)!
> - The resting intra-abdominal pressure is often increased up to 8–9 mmHg!

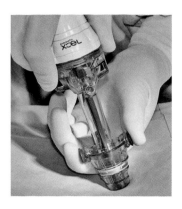

Size 11 scalpel
Scissors
2 surgical forceps
2 Langenbeck hooks
2 retaining sutures (2–0)
Purse-string suture (2–0)
Hasson trocar (10/12 mm)

In obese patients, the use of the Hasson technique can be very difficult or even impossible!

Incise the skin about a hand's breadth below the xiphoid and 1–2 fingers paramedian on the left, making a 3-cm skin incision.

Ensure that the skin incision is the correct length:
- **An incision that is too small can make the insertion of the trocars much more difficult. If the skin around the trocar then suffers increased tension, this may lead to skin necrosis!**
- **An incision that is too large can result in gas loss and trocar dislocation (→ p. 66, V-4b)!**

Spread the subcutaneous fat with the scissors as far as the rectus abdominis muscle. Use two Langenbeck hooks to expose the fascia of the anterior rectus sheath.

Then insert two 2-0 retaining sutures on the fascia of the anterior rectus sheath and draw the fascia upwards by pulling the sutures.

Use a scalpel to open the fascia between the two retaining sutures over a distance of 1.5 cm. Then spread the rectus abdominis muscle as far as the posterior rectus sheath.

To expose the fascia of the posterior rectus sheath, retract the rectus abdominis muscle with its anterior sheath by repositioning the Langenbeck hooks.

Now lift the fascia of the posterior rectus sheath and the peritoneum with the surgical forceps and incise them with the scissors over a length of about 1–1.5 cm. Check for the presence of close adhesions by inserting a finger into the incision site and palpating over the entire 360° circumference of the site.

Place a purse-string suture around the peritoneal incision and introduce the blunt Hasson trocar through the incision into the free abdominal cavity.

Secure the trocar with the two previously placed retaining sutures by tying them around the wings of the trocar cone. Tighten the purse-string suture around the Hasson trocar.

Secure the CO_2 supply tube to the trocar, remove the obturator, and insufflate the gas until the preselected maximum pressure of 12 mmHg is reached.

Alternative: It is possible to perform an open technique without using a Hasson trocar. After incising the fascia of the posterior rectus sheath and the peritoneum place a blunt probe through the incision in the free abdominal cavity, using it as a support for the placement of the trocar for the scope under visual control.

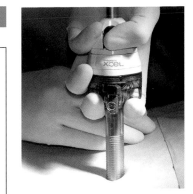

b) Trocar with optical obturator

Size 11 scalpel
Trocar with optical obturator
Scope (0°)

Incise the skin about a hand's breadth below the xiphoid and 1–2 fingers paramedian on the left, making a 1- to 1.5-cm skin incision.

Ensure that the skin incision is the correct length:
- **An incision that is too small can make the insertion of the trocars much more difficult. If the skin around the trocar then suffers increased tension, this may lead to skin necrosis!**
- **An incision that is too large can result in gas loss and trocar dislocation (→ p. 66, V-4b)!**

Insert the scope into the optical obturator located in the trocar and lock it.

Place the transparent conical tip into the incision. Now carefully push the different layers of the abdominal wall tangentially apart by applying light pressure and using to-and-fro rotating movements of the blunt obturator tip. The special construction of the obturator allows the layers to be identified before they are pushed apart.

Perform this tissue separation and the final perforation of the peritoneum under constant vision.

When inserting the trocar, take care
- **to go in perpendicular to the abdominal wall,**
- **to support the trocar with the hand, and**
- **not to use excessive force in order to avoid blood vessel and organ injuries in the event of loss of resistance (→ p. 65, V-2; V-3)!**

Finally, remove the scope together with the obturator from the trocar.

Secure the CO_2 supply tube to the trocar and insufflate the gas until the preselected maximum pressure of 12 mmHg is reached.

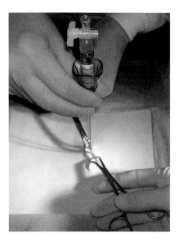

c) Veress needle (closed technique)

Insertion of the Veress needle and the first trocar are the most dangerous moments in minimally invasive surgery, as the insertion is done "blind". There are many reported cases of major injuries to the aorta and the iliac artery caused by the use of the Veress needle!

Size 11 scalpel
2 Backhaus clamps
Veress needle
10-ml syringe with NaCl solution
Trocar for the scope T1 (10/12 mm)

To minimize the risk of injury that may be caused by the Veress needle, select access in the left upper abdomen, subcostally in the midclavicular line.

In obese patients always select the access for the Veress needle in the left upper abdomen because of the usually existing hepatomegaly and the considerable amount of fatty tissue in these patients!

Patients who have undergone previous surgery carry a higher risk of having adhesions. In these patients or in case of hepatomegaly, the Veress needle should be used with caution!

Incise the skin about a hand's breadth below the xiphoid and 1–2 fingers paramedian on the left, making a 1- to 1.5-cm skin incision.

With the help of the assistant, elevate the abdominal wall with two Backhaus clamps, and carefully insert the Veress needle vertically, with your hand supported above the skin incision. The penetration of the abdominal wall layers by the Veress needle can be felt or even heard.

When inserting the Veress needle, take care
• to go in perpendicular to the abdominal wall (→ p. 66, V-4a),
• to support the hand holding the needle, and
• not to use excessive force in order to avoid blood vessel and organ injuries in the event of loss of resistance (→ p. 65, V-2; V-3)!

Check the correct position of the Veress needle by applying the following obligatory safety tests:

Aspiration test
Attach a 10-ml syringe filled with NaCl solution to the Veress needle. It should be possible to aspirate air as a sign that the intra-abdominal position is correct.

Injection test
Inject NaCl solution through the Veress needle into the abdominal cavity. This can be done easily if it is in the correct position. Increased resistance of the syringe plunger indicates a possible incorrect position of the Veress needle.

Alternative: When using the Endopath® Veress Needle Ultra (Ethicon Endo-Surgery), the valve is opened to perform the injection test, whereupon the NaCl solution is released into the abdominal cavity if the Veress needle is in the correct position. In addition, the red marker ball drops down, indicating that NaCl solution is being released into the abdominal cavity.

Rotation test

Carefully rotate the slightly tilted needle inside the abdominal cavity. If the needle can be rotated freely, adhesions in the close proximity are unlikely.

Slurp test

Notice that the slurp test is hardly feasible in case of pronounced obesity!

Apply one drop of NaCl solution onto the cone of the Veress needle, placing it convex on the opening. Now pull up the abdominal wall, making sure not to fix the Veress needle with your hand. Elevating the abdominal wall will create a partial vacuum, which in turn will cause the drop of NaCl to be sucked into the abdominal cavity, provided the Veress needle is correctly placed. A substantial vacuum will cause an additional "slurping" sound to be heard at the cone of the Veress needle.

If the safety tests indicate that the Veress needle has been placed correctly, attach the gas supply tube.

Excessively high intra-abdominal resting pressure and no flow indicate that the tip of the Veress needle is obstructed, e.g. by the greater omentum (→ **p. 65, V-3a**). In this case, perform the following test:

Manometer test

In order to release the Veress needle, manually lift up the abdominal wall. This should result in an obvious pressure drop. If this is not the case, remove the Veress needle and then place it again.

Notice that in obese patients the resting intra-abdominal pressure is often increased up to 8–9 mmHg!

Insufflate the CO_2 until the preselected maximum pressure of 12 mmHg is reached (recommended maximum flow through the Veress needle: ~1.8 l/min). After that, remove the Veress needle from the skin incision.

To be sure that the Veress needle has been placed correctly, check for an adequate flow during the CO_2 insufflation and for an appropriate increase in pressure on the insufflator!

Now place the trocar for the scope in the skin incision a hand's breadth below the xiphoid and 1–2 fingers paramedian on the left. To do so use either

- a trocar with a sharp tip (10/12 mm) or
- a trocar with optical obturator.

When inserting the trocar, take care
- **to go in perpendicular to the abdominal wall,**
- **to support the trocar with the hand, and**
- **not to use excessive force in order to avoid blood vessel and organ injuries in the event of loss of resistance (→ p. 65, V-2; V-3)!**

> Trocar for the scope T1 (10/12 mm)
> Working trocar T2 (5 mm or 10/12 mm; depending on the liver retracting device)
> Working trocar T3 (5 mm or 10/12 mm)
> Working trocar T4 (15 mm; for insertion of the gastric band)
> Size 11 scalpel
> Reducer caps, if necessary

Insert the scope into the trocar (T1).

Then position the patient in a 30° reverse Trendelenburg position in order to make the small intestine slide into the lower abdomen by gravity and to obtain an optimal view of the operating field (→ p. 22, I).

Perform a diagnostic laparoscopy to make sure that there are no pathological changes and/or injuries which might change the operative strategy or even prevent continuation of the operation (→ **p. 65, V-2; V-3**).

The liver is retracted through the trocar T2. The positions of the other working trocars depend on the operative site and are therefore established after the liver retracting device has been inserted.

Place the working trocar T2 subcostally on the right, approximately in the anterior axillary line. Choose the working trocar site T2 by palpating the abdominal wall under vision and use diaphanoscopy to ensure that no major cutaneous vessels will be injured when the trocar is inserted (→ **p. 65, V-1; V-2**).

> **T2:** In the right upper abdomen, subcostal, anterior axillary line (depending on liver size and liver retracting device)

Incise the skin with a scalpel according to the trocar diameter: about 1 cm when using a 5-mm trocar and 1.5 cm with a 10/12-mm trocar. Now insert the working trocar under vision.

Ensure that the skin incision is the right size!

When placing the trocar make sure that it points exactly towards the operating field, as later corrections will not be possible.

When placing the trocar, take care
- **to insert the trocar under vision to avoid injuries (→ p. 65, V-2; V-3), and**
- **to point the trocar exactly towards the operating field, as later corrections will be difficult, if not impossible in obese abdominal walls!**

After the liver retracting device has been inserted, an unrestricted view of the operating field should be guaranteed. Then fix the liver retracting device to the fixation arm.

Place the liver retracting device carefully and always under vision, as in obese patients the texture of the liver is often fat, which increases the vulnerability of the tissue (→ p. 66, V-3d)!

Choose the working trocar sites T3 and T4 depending on the operative site, roughly in a half-moon around the trocar for the scope, and by palpating the abdominal wall under vision. Use diaphanoscopy to ensure that no major cutaneous vessels will be injured when the trocar is inserted (→ **p. 65, V-1; V-2**).

> **T3:** In the right epigastrium, depending on liver size
>
> **T4:** In the left epigastrium, subcostal, midclavicular line

Insert the trocars according to the above description for T2, starting with the skin incisions. For the 15-mm trocar (T4) make a 3- to 3.5-cm skin incision with a scalpel.

> **When placing the trocars, take care**
> • to insert the trocars under vision to avoid injuries (→ p. 65, V-2; V-3),
> • to point the trocars exactly towards the operating field, as later corrections will be difficult, if not impossible in obese abdominal walls,
> • to place additional trocars at any time to gain optimal working conditions, and
> • to place the trocars with a minimum distance of 10 cm between them in order to avoid interference from scope and instruments!

Remove the obturators from the trocars and attach the reducer caps to T3 and T4, if necessary.

> **Alternative:** If the liver is greatly enlarged, requiring the use of another liver retracting device, insert an additional trocar (T5). The location of the trocar depends on the intra-operative site.

> There are many ways to position the trocars. We prefer the following placement, but it should be the surgeon's choice!

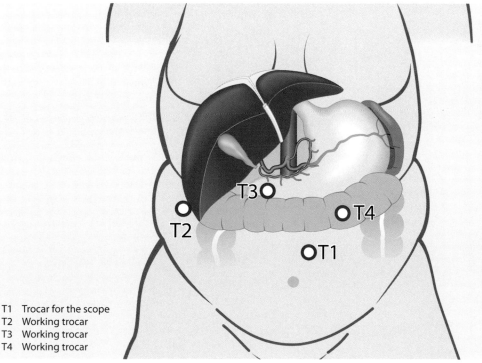

T1 Trocar for the scope
T2 Working trocar
T3 Working trocar
T4 Working trocar

01 Exploring the abdominal cavity

02 Identifying the anatomical landmarks

03 Dissecting the pars flaccida

04 Dissecting the angle of His

05 Introducing the gastric band

06 Creating the retrocardial tunnel and connecting the gastric band with the Goldfinger™

07 Positioning the gastric band

08 Closing the gastric band

09 Placing the safety sutures

10 Testing the stomach for leaks

11 Inspecting the operating field and removing the trocars

12 Attaching and fixing the port system – Velocity™

13 Finishing the operation

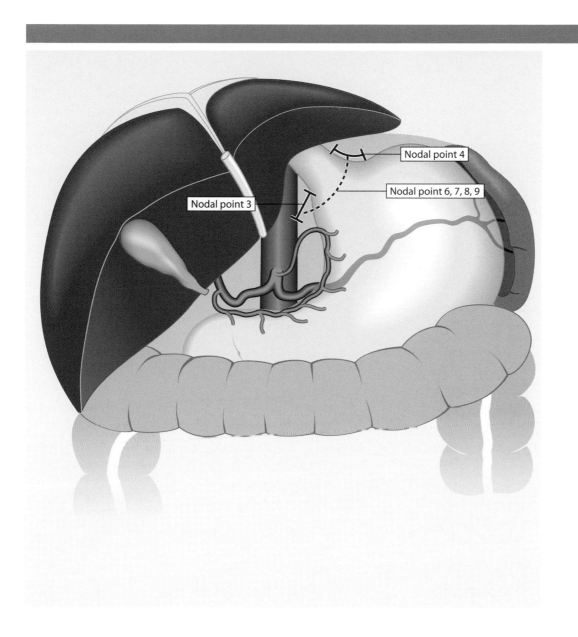

Nodal point 4

Nodal point 6, 7, 8, 9

Nodal point 3

1 Exploring the abdominal cavity

T1 Scope
T2 Liver retracting device
T3 Atraumatic grasping forceps, if necessary
T4 HF electrode or curved scissors, if necessary

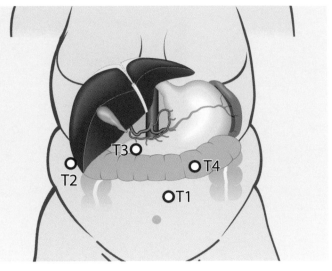

Examine the abdominal cavity carefully by inspecting it in a clockwise direction. Due to obesity a thorough inspection of the structures in the pelvis might be difficult.

- Pelvis: dome of the urinary bladder, pouch of Douglas, the internal hernial orifices, and the uterus and adnexa in women
- Cecum with appendix
- Ascending colon
- Right upper abdomen: liver and gallbladder, right colonic flexure
- Greater omentum
- Transverse colon
- Left upper abdomen: stomach and spleen, splenic flexure
- Descending colon
- Sigmoid colon
- Jejunum and ileum

Look particularly for adhesions, erythema, vascular injections, serous fluid, pus, tumors and peritoneal carcinosis.

If a tumor or an infection is found, implantation of the gastric band is contraindicated!

Check the trocar incision sites particularly for adhesions and possible bleedings. Change the scope position, if necessary (→ **p. 65, V-1; V-2**).

Divide any adhesions in the operating field using sharp dissection (→ **p. 65, V-1**).

Divide any adhesions to organs promptly in order to avoid injuries (→ p. 65, V-3)!

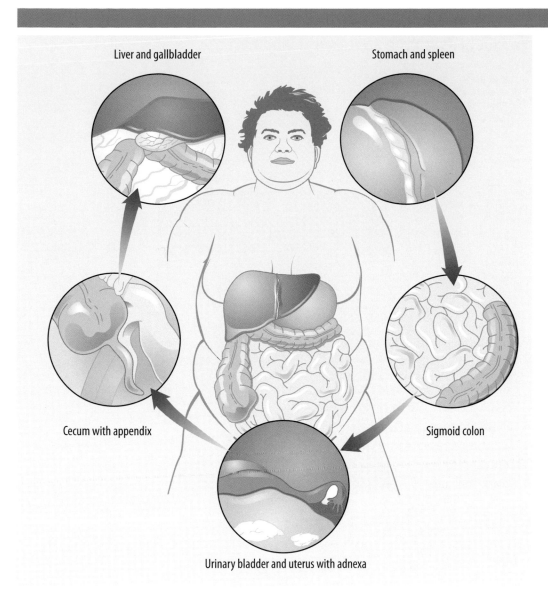

Liver and gallbladder

Stomach and spleen

Cecum with appendix

Sigmoid colon

Urinary bladder and uterus with adnexa

2 Identifying the anatomical landmarks

T1   Scope
T2   Liver retracting device
T3   Atraumatic grasping forceps
T4   Curved dissector,
        HF electrode or curved
        scissors, if necessary

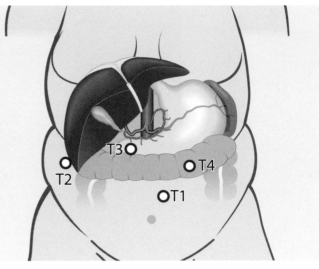

Identify the following anatomical landmarks:

Upper abdomen:
- Caudate and left liver lobe with falciform ligament
- Lesser omentum with hepatogastric ligament
- Left gastric artery
- Gastro-esophageal junction
- Stomach: lesser and greater curvature, angle of His
- Spleen with gastrophrenic ligament

In case of fat accumulations in the subcardiac region of the stomach and at the gastro-esophageal junction, use a curved dissector or sharp dissection to remove them in order to ensure an optimal view of the operating field.

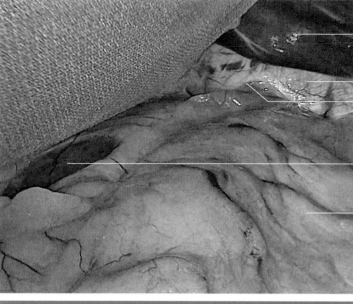

Liver

Diaphragm

Hiatus esophagus

Caudate liver lobe

Stomach

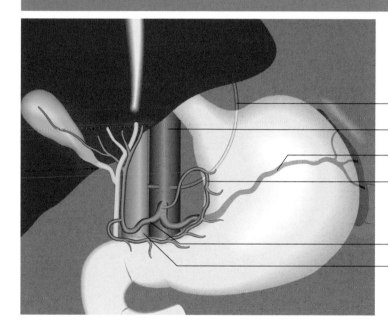

Inferior phrenic artery

Aorta

Splenic artery

Left gastric artery

Common hepatic artery

Vena cava

3 Dissecting the pars flaccida

T1   Scope
T2   Liver retracting device
T3   Atraumatic grasping forceps
T4   HF electrode

– Gastric calibration tube
– 30-ml syringe
– 25 ml saline solution, if necessary

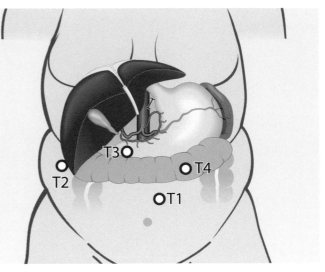

Ask the anesthetist to pass the gastric calibration tube into the stomach and to slowly fill the balloon of the tube with 25 ml saline solution or air. Then tell him to draw the tube back until the balloon comes by the gastro-esophageal junction in order to determine its location precisely (→ **p. 65, V-3b; p. 66, V-3c**).

Grasp the lesser omentum with the atraumatic grasping forceps (T3) to stretch the pars flaccida.

Incise the pars flaccida caudal to the gastro-esophageal junction and cranial to the left gastric artery, making an approximately 5-cm incision with the HF electrode (T4). It is mandatory to incise the pars flaccida cranial to the left gastric artery in order not to open the omental bursa and thus to prevent a pouch dilatation.

> **Take care to perform the incision cranial to the left gastric artery in order not to open the omental bursa and thus to prevent a pouch dilatation (→ p. 67, V-6; p. 75, pouch dilatation)!**

While incising the pars flaccida, carefully identify the left gastric artery, the inferior phrenic artery, any accessory hepatic artery, and the branches of the vagal nerve located in this area.

> **Pay attention to the left gastric artery, the inferior phrenic artery, any accessory hepatic artery, and the branches of the vagal nerve in order to avoid any injuries (→ p. 65, V-2; p. 70, anatomical variations)!**

Expose the right crus of the diaphragm close to the gastro-esophageal junction. To create the entry of the retrocardial tunnel, incise the fatty tissue medial to the right crus of the diaphragm 0.5 cm in length and 5 cm distal to the gastro-esophageal junction with the HF electrode (T4). Be careful not to touch the diaphragm with the HF electrode in order not to provoke contractions.

> **Take care not to touch the diaphragm with the HF electrode, as this can provoke contractions possibly leading to blood vessel and organ injuries caused by the instruments (→ p. 65, V-2; V-3)!**

Ask the anesthetist to advance the calibration tube into the stomach.

Incising the pars flaccida

Liver retracting device

Caudate liver lobe

Pars flaccida

Stomach

Incising medial to the right crus of the diaphragm

Caudate liver lobe

Stomach

Right crus of the diaphragm

The later retrocardial tunnel

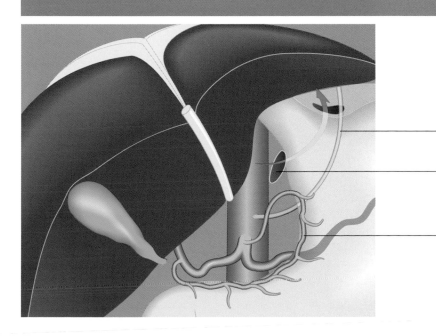

Inferior phrenic artery

Incised pars flaccida

Left gastric artery

4 Dissecting the angle of His

T1   Scope
T2   Liver retracting device
T3   Atraumatic grasping forceps
T4   HF electrode

– Gastric calibration tube

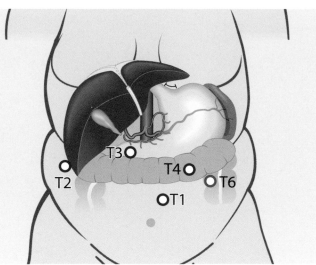

Grasp the gastric fundus with the atraumatic grasping forceps (T3) and pull it caudally to achieve excellent exposure of the angle of His.

To assure the later placement of the gastric band within the gastrophrenic ligament, incise the avascular part of the ligament at the angle of His over a distance of about 1 cm with the HF electrode in T4. Dissect in the direction of the right crus of the diaphragm and of the incised pars flaccida to create an exit for the later retrocardial tunnel.

Make sure to dissect in the direction of the right crus of the diaphragm and of the incised pars flaccida to prepare an exit for the later retrocardial tunnel!

Then expose the left crus of the diaphragm over a distance of 1–1.5 cm with the HF electrode (T4). While dissecting, pay attention not to injure the inferior phrenic artery, the short gastric veins and the vessels located in the left crus of the diaphragm, and be careful not to touch the diaphragm with the HF electrode in order not to provoke contractions.

Take care not to injure the inferior phrenic artery, the short gastric veins and the vessels located in the left crus of the diaphragm and not to touch the diaphragm with the HF electrode, as this can provoke contractions possibly leading to blood vessel and organ injuries caused by the instruments (→ p. 65, V-2; V-3)!

Alternative: If the view of the angle of His is limited, introduce an additional 5-mm trocar (T6) subcostally in the anterior axillary line beneath and left-lateral of T4 in the left upper abdomen quadrant. Introduce an atraumatic grasping forceps in T6 and draw the greater omentum caudally for excellent exposure of the angle of His.

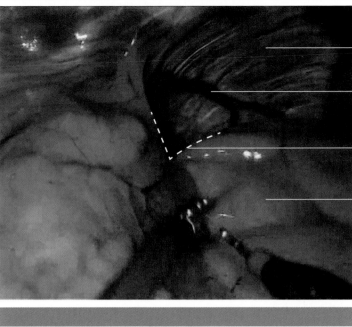

Diaphragm

Inferior phrenic artery

Angle of His

Stomach

Incising the gastrophrenic ligament at the angle of His

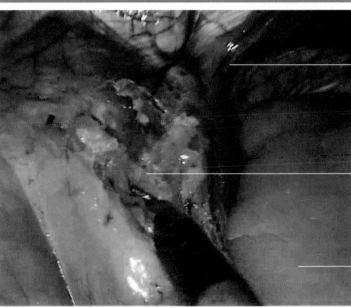

Inferior phrenic artery

Gastrophrenic ligament

Stomach

Correct incision above the omental bursa

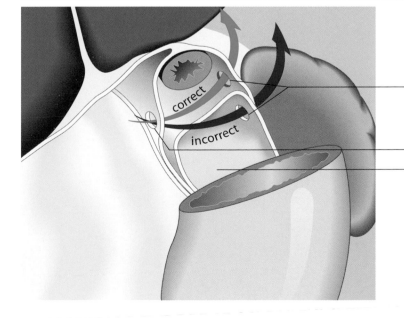

Incised gastrophrenic ligament

Incised pars flaccida
Omental bursa

5 Introducing the gastric band

T1   Scope
T2   Liver retracting device
T3   –
T4   Atraumatic grasping forceps
     with SAGB Gastric Band

– Gastric calibration tube

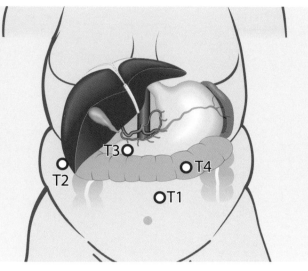

Carefully inspect and check the band prepared by the scrub nurse (→ p. 21, I)!

Grasp the gastric band with the atraumatic grasping forceps at its band extender flap directly behind the pre-lock flanges. It is mandatory to position the balloon of the band along the forceps shaft in order to prevent damage to the balloon inside the trocar valve.

Take care not to grasp the balloon with any instruments, as this may result in damage to the balloon, and to position the gastric band with the balloon along the forceps shaft to prevent damage to the band inside the trocar valve!

Under vision introduce the atraumatic grasping forceps together with the gastric band into the abdominal cavity through the 15-mm trocar (T4), accepting a slight loss of gas.

Pass the atraumatic grasping forceps with the gastric band through the 15-mm trocar (T4) under vision in order to avoid damage to the gastric band and blood vessel and organ injuries (→ p. 65, V-2; V-3).

Then insert the complete tubing system into the abdominal cavity with the atraumatic grasping forceps (T4).

Re-establish the pneumoperitoneum if necessary.

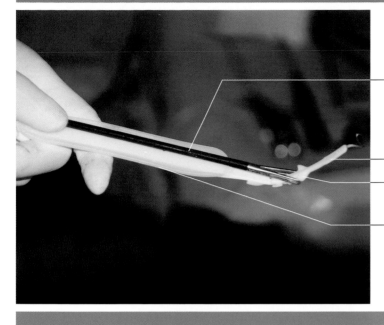

Atraumatic grasping forceps

Band extender

Pre-lock flanges

Balloon

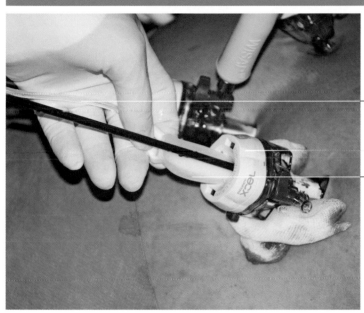

Tubing

15-mm trocar

Balloon

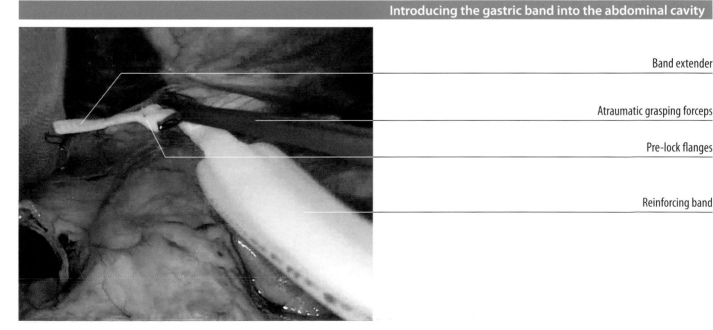

Band extender

Atraumatic grasping forceps

Pre-lock flanges

Reinforcing band

6 Creating the retrocardial tunnel and connecting the gastric band with the Goldfinger™

T1   Scope
T2   Liver retracting device
T3   Goldfinger™
T4   Atraumatic grasping forceps, later dissecting swab, if necessary, later curved dissector

– SAGB Gastric Band
– Gastric calibration tube
– 30-ml syringe

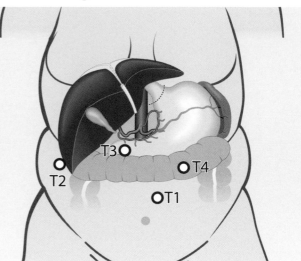

Introduce the Goldfinger™ through T3. Form its distal tip into a slight curve. Check the curvature of the Goldfinger™ in front of the anterior wall of the stomach so that it corresponds to the later retrocardial course of the tunnel.

Grasp the gastric fundus with the atraumatic grasping forceps (T4) and pull it caudomedially.

Then gently introduce the Goldfinger™, starting from the incision at the right crus of the diaphragm retrocardially towards the incision at the angle of His until the tip of the Goldfinger™ appears there. Guide the Goldfinger™ with caution to avoid injuries to the stomach or the esophagus, and be careful not to deviate from the plane of dissection to ensure a small pouch size of about 15 ml.

Guide the Goldfinger™ with caution to avoid injuries to the stomach or the esophagus, and take care not to deviate from the plane of dissection to ensure a small pouch size of about 15 ml (→ p. 65, V-3b; p. 66, V-3c; p. 75, pouch dilatation)!

In case of any resistance on moving the Goldfinger™ forward, re-check its position and use a dissecting swab (T4) to wipe the connective tissue from its tip or remove and replace the Goldfinger™, starting again from the right crus of the diaphragm. If there is the slightest suspicion of a perforation, test the stomach for leaks at once.

If there is the slightest suspicion of a perforation, test the stomach for leaks at once (→ p. 52, nodal point 10; p. 66, V-3c)!

Hook the suture loop of the gastric band into the notch of the Goldfinger™ using the curved dissector in T4.

Ask the anesthetist to empty the balloon of the gastric calibration tube fully and to withdraw it carefully into the esophagus (→ p. 65, V-3b).

Introducing the Goldfinger™ into the retrocardial space

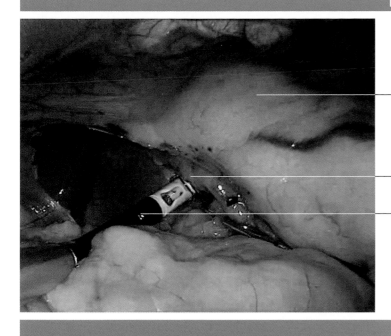

Stomach

Medial incision at the right crus of the diaphragm

Goldfinger™

Placing the Goldfinger™ into the retrocardial tunnel

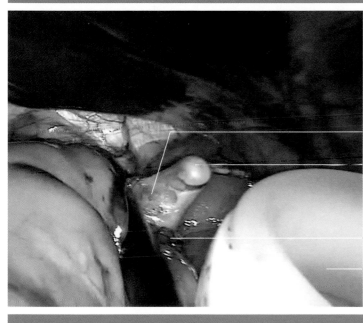

Connective tissue

Goldfinger™

Incision at the angle of His

SAGB Gastric Band

Connecting the gastric band with the Goldfinger™

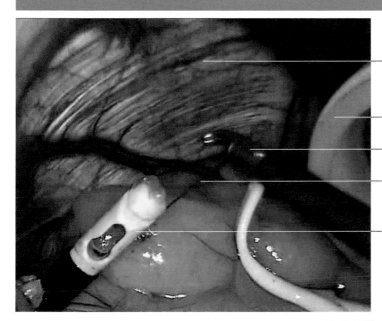

Diaphragm

SAGB Gastric Band

Curved dissector

Suture loop

Goldfinger™

7 Positioning the gastric band

T1   Scope
T2   Liver retracting device
T3   Goldfinger™, later atraumatic grasping forceps
T4   Curved dissector

– SAGB Gastric Band
– Gastric calibration tube

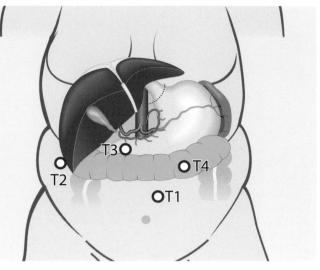

While pulling the gastric band through the retrocardial tunnel make sure to position the gastric band so that its balloon is oriented towards the stomach wall.

> **Pay attention to position the gastric band in the retrocardial tunnel so that its balloon is oriented towards the stomach wall!**

Pull the Goldfinger™ with the attached band under vision slowly and carefully from the angle of His through the retrocardial tunnel until the band extender flap appears at the lesser curvature. Use the curved dissector (T4) to assist the sliding of the band through the tunnel.

If excessive resistance is noticed while pulling the gastric band through the tunnel, check the adequacy of the retrocardial tissue dissection and extend dissection if necessary.

> **Do not pull the band against excessive resistance through the tunnel in order to avoid injuries. If excessive resistance is noticed, check the adequacy of the retrocardial tissue dissection and extend dissection if necessary (→ p. 66, V-3c)!**

Grasp the extender flap of the band on the side of the lesser curvature with the curved dissector (T4), then remove the Goldfinger™ carefully in order to avoid dislocation of the gastric band and any injury to the liver.

> **To avoid dislocation of the retrocardially positioned gastric band and any injury to the liver, remove the Goldfinger™ from the abdominal cavity with care (→ p. 66, V-3d)!**

Introduce the atraumatic grasping forceps through T3 and grasp the extender flap of the band to pull the entire gastric band through the tunnel. Then check the correct position of the band.

In case the band is not in the correct position, re-grasp the band extender flap on the lesser curvature side with the atraumatic grasping forceps (T3) and rotate the instrument around its long axis until the balloon lies adjacent to the posterior wall of the stomach.

SAGB Gastric Band

Stomach

Band extender

Suture loop

Goldfinger™

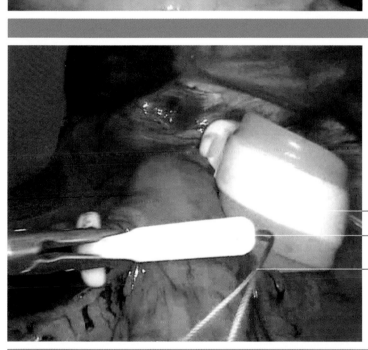

SAGB Gastric Band

Band extender

Suture loop

Correct positioning of the gastric band

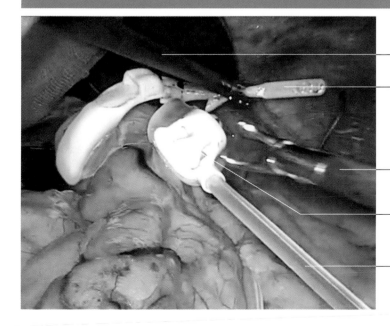

Atraumatic grasping forceps

Band extender

Curved dissector

Buckle tab

Tubing

8 Closing the gastric band

T1 Scope
T2 Liver retracting device
T3 Atraumatic grasping forceps
T4 Curved dissector, later curved
     scissors, later atraumatic
     grasping forceps

– SAGB Gastric Band
– Gastric calibration tube

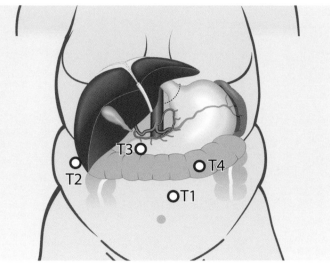

To close the gastric band, grasp its band extender flap directly behind the pre-lock flanges with the atraumatic grasping forceps in T3. Then grasp the buckle tab with the curved dissector (T4) and draw the band extender through the buckle until the pre-lock flanges pass through the buckle.

Re-grasp the band extender flap with the curved dissector (T4) and the buckle tab with the atraumatic grasping forceps (T3) and pull the locking shell on the buckle tongue to lock the band. Then cut the extender strap at the black cutting indicator with curved scissors (T4) and remove the band extender with the atraumatic grasping forceps (T4).

When closing the gastric band, take care not to draw any part of the stomach or fatty tissue into the band fastening and not to close the band too tightly around the stomach.

> When closing the gastric band, make sure that no tissue is trapped in the band fastening and that the band is not closed too tightly (→ p. 66, V-3c; p. 67, V-7)!

Ensure not to damage the balloon with any instrument and to maintain the band in its correct retrocardial position.

> Ensure that the balloon is not damaged by the instruments and that the band maintains its correct retrocardial position (→ p. 75, pouch dilatation)!

Finally, check the correct position and the tightness of the gastric band. If the band is positioned incorrectly or is too tight, re-open the band at its fastening and close it again properly as described above or use the combined technique (→ p. 67, V-7).

> Pay attention that the gastric band is in the correct position and not too tight around the stomach before continuing with the operation!

Closing the gastric band

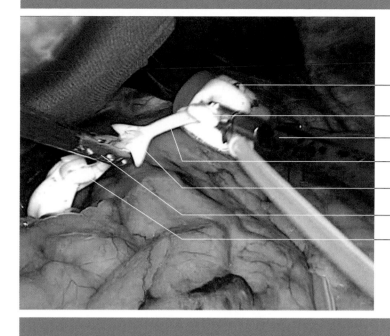

Buckle tongue

Buckle tab

Curved dissector

Band extender

Pre-lock flanges

Atraumatic grasping forceps

Extender strap

Locking the gastric band

Locking shell

Band extender

Buckle tongue including lock indicator

Buckle tab

Curved dissector

Atraumatic grasping forceps

Tubing

Checking the correct position of the gastric band

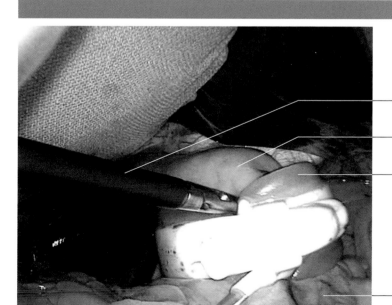

Atraumatic grasping forceps

Pouch

SAGB Gastric Band

Stomach

9 Placing the safety sutures

T1   Scope
T2   Liver retracting device
T3   Atraumatic grasping forceps, later curved scissors
T4   Needle holder

– Safety sutures 2–0 non-absorbable, polyfilament
– SAGB Gastric Band
– Gastric calibration tube

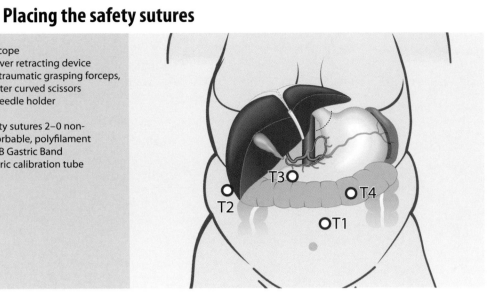

Before placing the safety sutures, draw the fastening of the band in the direction of the lesser curvature with the atraumatic grasping forceps (T3).

With the first suture, fix the fundus of the stomach to the left crus of the diaphragm in order to keep the gastric band in its correct position (→ p. 75, band complications).

Place two additional sutures anteriorly between the fundus and the pouch in order to surround the band completely by a cuff of stomach wall. It is important to sew the complete seromuscular layer of the stomach wall.

> **When placing the safety sutures take care to sew the complete seromuscular layer of the stomach wall!**

Make sure that the band fastening remains freely accessible for later revisions and that the cuff is not too tight and will allow subsequent unrestricted inflation of the balloon during adjustment of the gastric band. If in doubt, perform a trial filling of the band.

> **Pay attention that the band fastening remains freely accessible after placing the sutures and that the cuff is not too tight and will allow subsequent unrestricted filling of the gastric band (→ p. 73, band adjustment)!**

In order not to damage the gastric band, position the safety sutures under vision and avoid direct contact between the sutures and the gastric band.

> **To avoid damage to the gastric band, take care to have the needle under vision when positioning the safety sutures close to the band and to have no direct contact between the sutures and the gastric band!**

Re-check the correct position of the gastric band.

> **Alternative: If the gastric band fits properly on the gastro-esophageal junction and cannot slip, perform only the first safety suture (fundus to left crus of diaphragm) and no gastro-gastric sutures.**

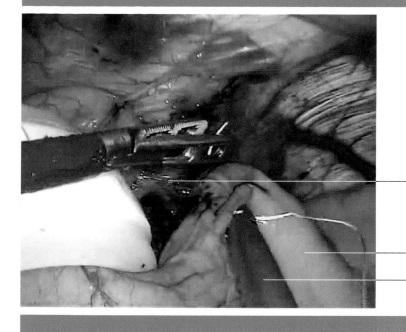

Left crus of the diaphragm

Fundus

Needle holder

Placing the second safety suture

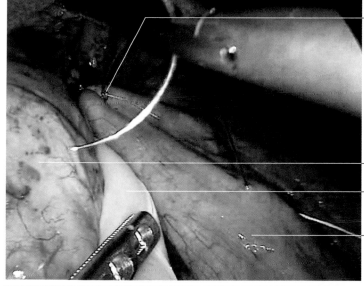

First safety suture

Pouch

SAGB Gastric Band

Fundus

Placing the third safety suture

Liver

First safety suture

Needle holder

Fundus

Pouch

10 Testing the stomach for leaks

T1   Scope
T2   Liver retracting device
T3   Atraumatic grasping forceps
T4   Atraumatic grasping forceps

– SAGB Gastric Band
– Gastric calibration tube
– Bowl with 20 ml methylene blue
  solution (5 ml methylene blue
  1 % with 15 ml saline solution)
– 10-ml syringe

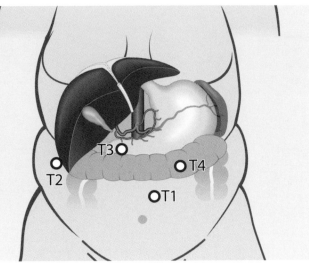

Note that a methylene blue test is a security check and does not guarantee that the stomach has not been injured! If in doubt, perform intraoperative gastroscopy (→ p. 66, V-3c)!

Ask the anesthetist to advance the gastric calibration tube carefully into the pouch just in front of the gastric band and have it filled with 20 ml methylene blue solution.

Check carefully whether methylene blue solution emerges anywhere on the stomach due to a hitherto unnoticed injury. Pay special attention to the poorly visible posterior wall of the stomach (→ **p. 66, V-3c**).

Then ask the anesthetist to suck off the liquid from the pouch and to remove the gastric calibration tube.

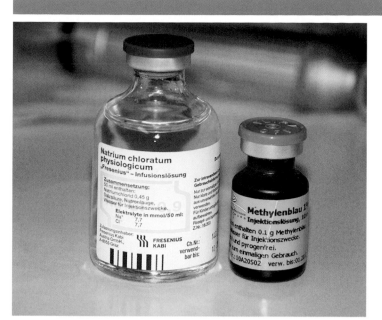

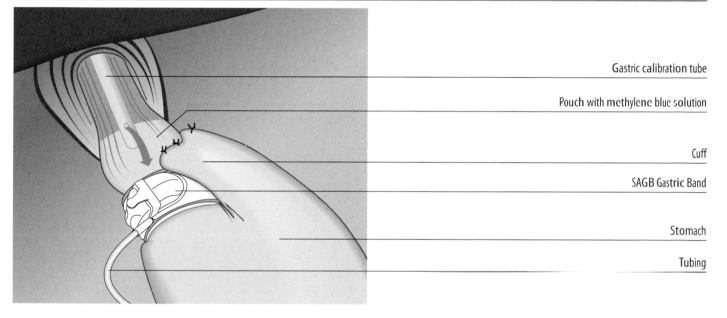

Gastric calibration tube

Pouch with methylene blue solution

Cuff

SAGB Gastric Band

Stomach

Tubing

11   Inspecting the operating field and removing the trocars

T1   Scope
T2   Liver retracting device
T3   Atraumatic grasping forceps
T4   HF electrode, if necessary, later atraumatic grasping forceps

– Surgical forceps
– Needle holder
– Suture scissors
– 2 Langenbeck hooks
– Fascia sutures 2–0 absorbable, polyfilament

– SAGB Gastric Band
– Trocar side closure device, if necessary

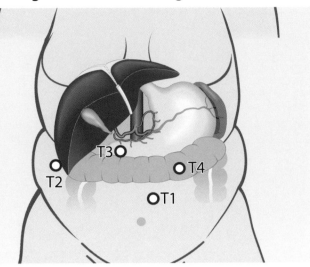

Inspect the operating field carefully and check for any bleeding and possible organ injuries. Stop any visible bleeding with the HF electrode (T4) and treat any organ injury before continuing the operation.

Make sure to stop any visible bleeding in the operative field in order to avoid postoperative bleeding and to treat any organ injury before continuing the operation (→ p. 65, V-2; V-3)!

Grasp the end of the tubing of the gastric band with the atraumatic grasping forceps (T4) and pull it out through T4 for the extracorporeal attachment of the port. Cut the tubing at its distal end to remove the one-way valve. Do not shorten the tubing in order to be able to treat a possibly occurring leakage from the tubing system or a port infection postoperatively by shortening and, in the latter case, by closing the tubing system.

It is recommended not to shorten the tubing when removing the one-way valve to be able to treat a possibly occurring leakage from the tubing system and port infection postoperatively (→ p. 77, leakage from the band system; port infection)!

Remove the 15-mm working trocar T4 carefully under vision in order not to damage the tubing system by excessive tension. Check the trocar incision with regard to possible bleeding.

Take care to remove the 15-mm working trocar T4 carefully in order not to damage the tubing system by excessive tension and check the trocar incision with regard to possible bleeding (→ p. 65, V-2)!

Close the fascia of the T4 entry site accurately with an absorbable suture to prevent possible hernia formation. Take care not to damage the tubing of the gastric band.

Pay attention not to damage the tubing system when closing the fascia of T4!

In case of heavier bleeding at the T4 entry site, close its fascia using a special trocar side closure device.

Remove the working trocars T2 and T3 under vision. Check the trocar incision for possible bleeding (→ **p. 65, V-2**).

Remove the scope and open the valve on the trocar for the scope (T1) for deflation. Then remove the trocar for the scope.

Inspecting the operating field

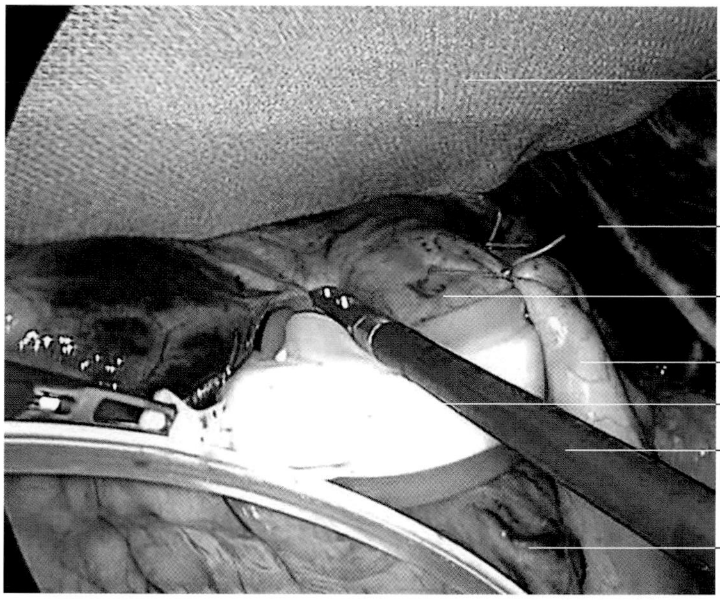
Liver retracting device
Liver
Pouch
Cuff
SAGB Gastric Band
Atraumatic grasping forceps
Stomach

Pulling out the tubing of the gastric band

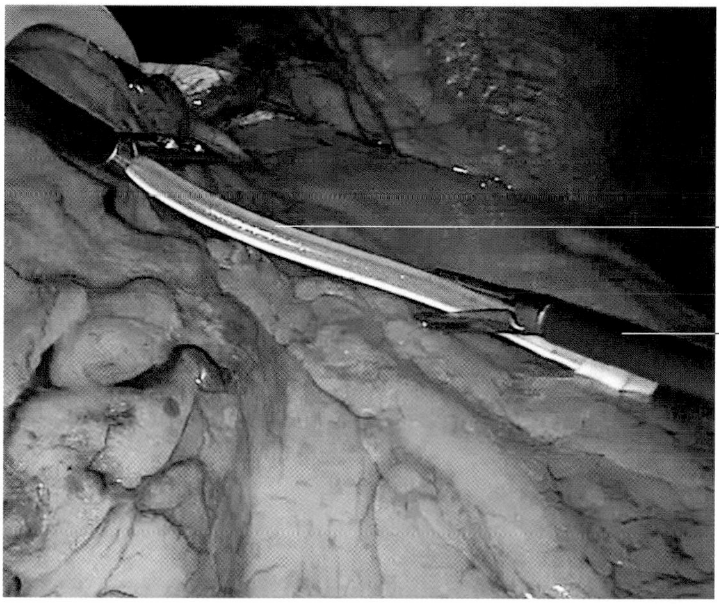
Tubing
Atraumatic grasping forceps

Cutting the tubing at its distal end

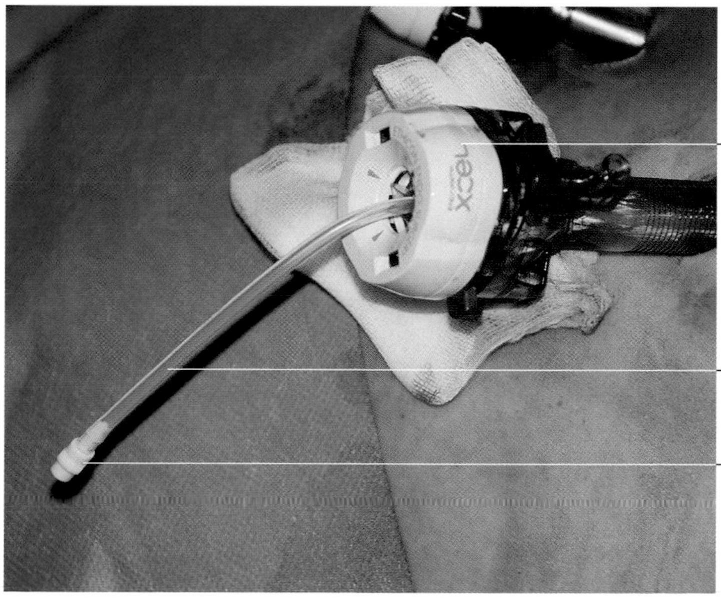
15-mm trocar
Tubing
One-way valve

12 Attaching and fixing the port system – Velocity™

T1 –
T2 –
T3 –
T4 Velocity™

– Surgical forceps
– Dissecting scissors
– 2 Langenbeck hooks
– Huber needle

– SAGB Gastric Band

The Velocity™ Injection Port is compatible ONLY with the Swedish Adjustable Gastric Bands manufactured by Obtech Medical, Ethicon Endo-Surgery!

Pay attention to place the port in a position on the patient where it can readily be located and accessed for band adjustments and where port migration and/or rotation will be prevented (→ p. 77, port rotation)!

Position two Langenbeck hooks at the skin incision of T4 to open it.

Dissect the fat completely away from the fascia of the anterior rectus sheath of T4 with dissecting scissors and create a fat-free space in order to place the port completely flat on the fascia. Then remove the two Langenbeck hooks.

Take care to place the port completely flat on the fascia of the anterior rectus sheath in order to avoid infection and penetration of the port (→ p. 77, port infection; port penetration)!

Slide the strain relief end of the locking connector onto the cut end of the tubing of the SAGB Gastric Band. Then push the tubing onto the connection tube extending from the port until the tubing has reached the outer face of the connection housing on the port.

With its tab facing upwards, slide the locking connector completely into the connection housing until the locking connector tab aligns with the notch in the connection housing of the port.

Make sure that the locking connector tab aligns with the notch in the connection housing of the port to enable the locking connector to slide into the connection housing in the next step!

Turn the locking connector clockwise until the connector stops rotating and the locking connector tab lies completely in the notch of the connection housing. Resistance may be felt and there may be an audible click.

Aspirate air from the port using a Huber needle. Use only a Huber needle to avoid injuries to the septum of the injection port.

To avoid injuries to the septum of the injection port, use only a Huber needle to aspirate air!

Pushing the tubing onto the connection tube

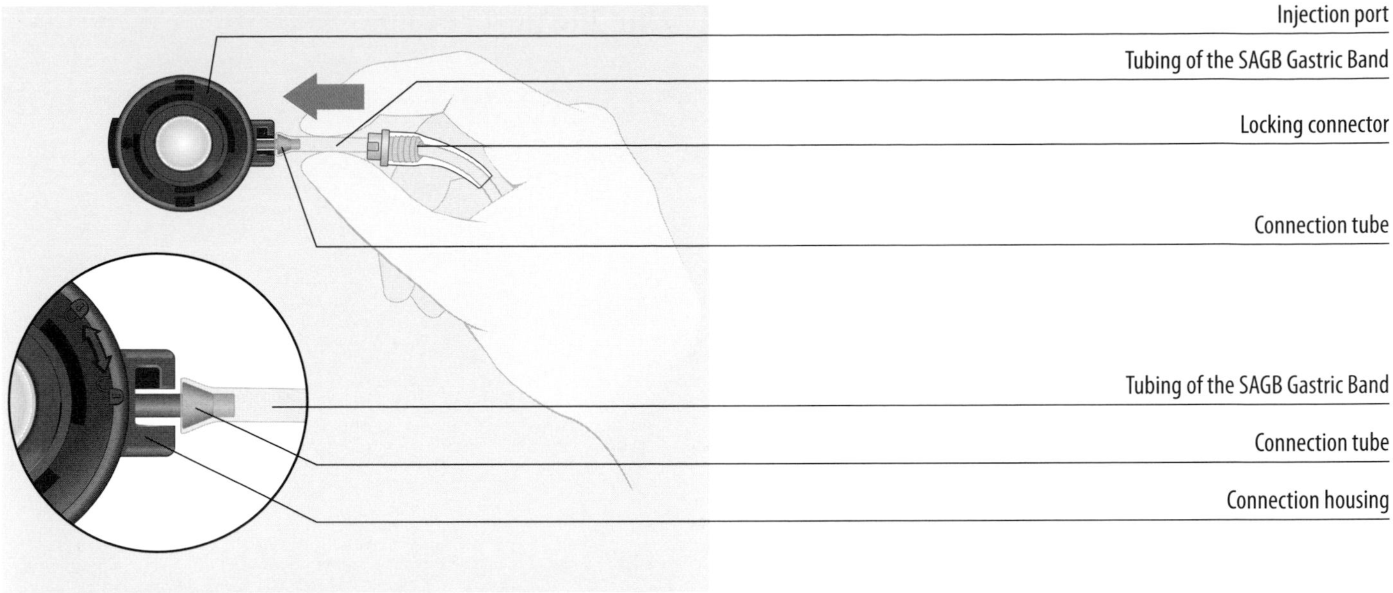

Injection port

Tubing of the SAGB Gastric Band

Locking connector

Connection tube

Tubing of the SAGB Gastric Band

Connection tube

Connection housing

Sliding the locking connector into the connection housing

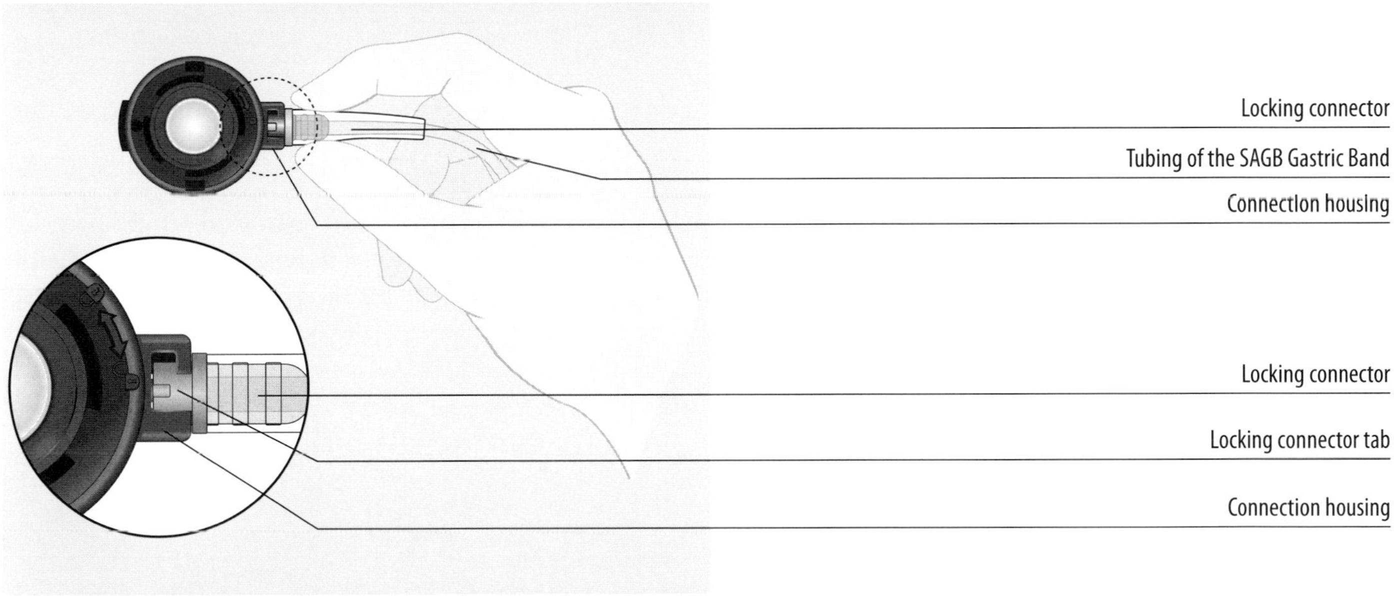

Locking connector

Tubing of the SAGB Gastric Band

Connection housing

Locking connector

Locking connector tab

Connection housing

Turning the locking connector clockwise

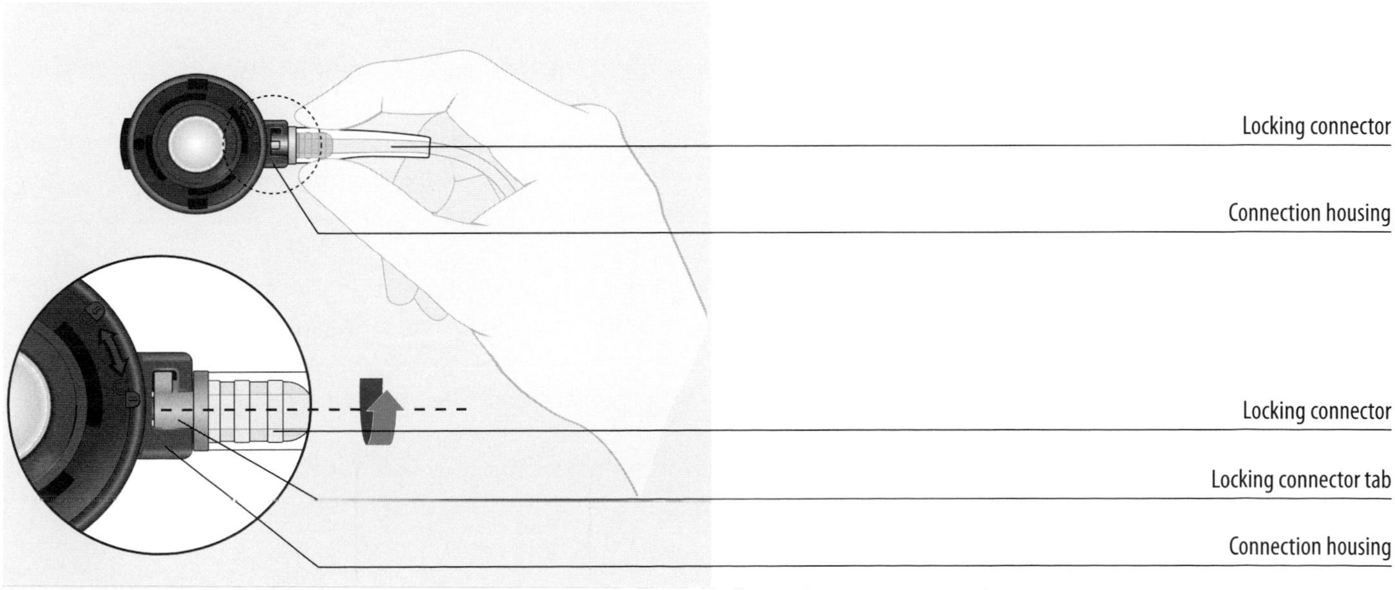

Locking connector

Connection housing

Locking connector

Locking connector tab

Connection housing

12 Attaching and fixing the port system – Velocity™

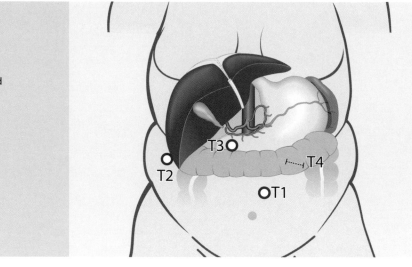

```
T1   –
T2   –
T3   –
T4   Velocity™

–  SAGB Gastric Band
```

Check the port to ensure that the actuator ring is in the unlocked position. In the unlocked position the fastening hooks are retracted into the port and are not exposed. If the actuator ring is not in the unlocked position, rotate it counter-clockwise to position it in the unlocked position.

Make sure that the actuator ring is in the unlocked position before inserting it into the applier receptacle!

With the tubing connected and the actuator ring in the unlocked position, insert the port with attached red safety cap into the applier receptacle. Make sure that the safety cap is facing opposite the applier and that the connection housing fits into one of the two guide notches. The port will snap into place in the applier.

Pay attention that the red safety cap is facing opposite the applier and the connection housing fits into one of the two guide notches when inserting the port into the applier receptacle!

Remove the safety cap from the bottom of the port.

Then grasp the handle of the port applier in the palm of one hand. It is important not to depress the red safety release trigger accidentally in order to avoid early release.

Take care not to depress the red safety release trigger in order to avoid early release!

Insert the applier receptacle at an angle with the tubing and locking connector entering the incision first and place the port on the prepared fascia. When inserting the applier receptacle, pay attention not to kink the band tubing.

Take care to avoid kinks in the band tubing when inserting the applier receptacle with the port (→ p. 79, disconnection of the port and tubing system)!

Apply light downward pressure to the applier to make the port rest completely flat on the fascia.

Excessive downward pressure is not necessary to achieve satisfactory attachment of the port to the tissue and may reduce the ability of the port to attach adequately!

Checking the unlocked position of the actuator ring

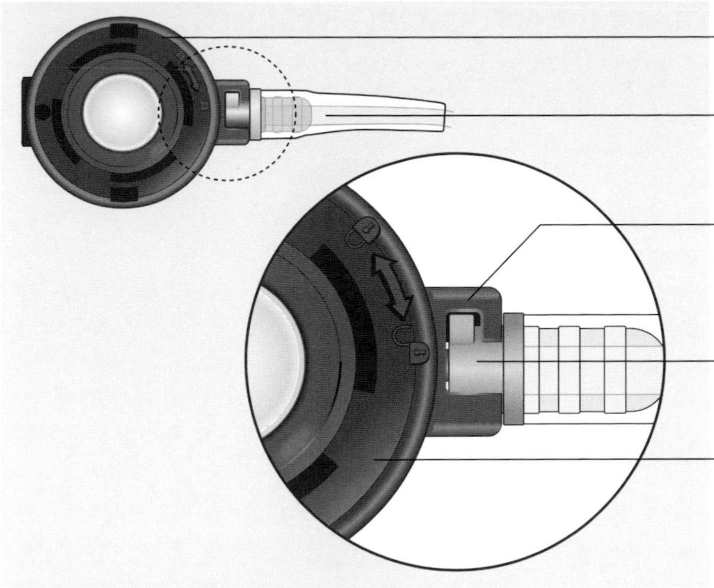

Actuator ring

Locking connector

Connection housing

Locking connector tab

Actuator ring in unlocked position

Inserting the port into the applier receptacle

Applier receptacle

Guide notch

Injection port

Safety cap

Locking connector

Tubing of the SAGB Gastric Band

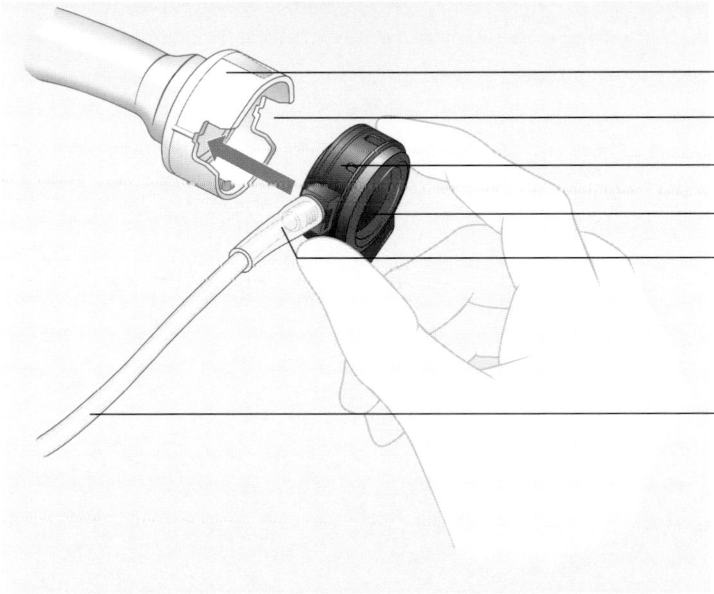

Inserting the applier receptacle

Firing lever

Handle

Port applier

Safety release trigger

Applier shaft

Applier receptacle with injection port

Skin incision

Tubing of the SAGB Gastric Band

Fascia

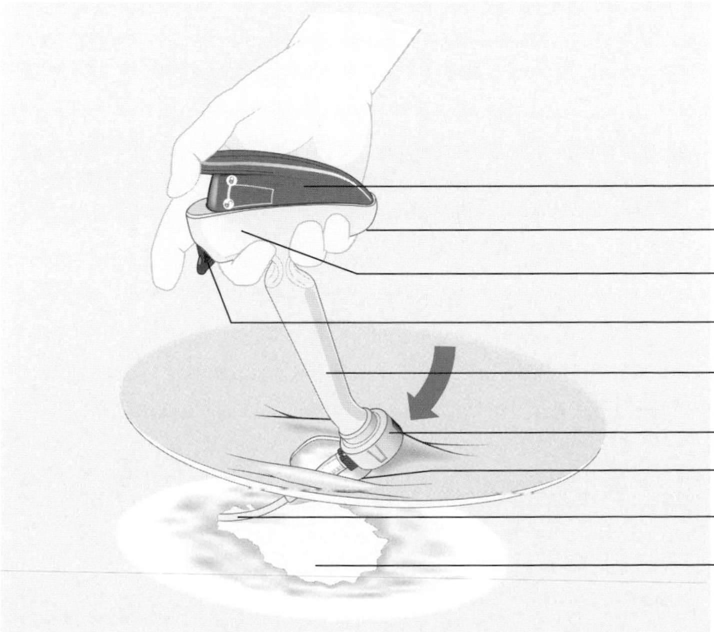

NODAL POINTS

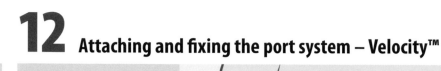

12 Attaching and fixing the port system – Velocity™

T1 –
T2 –
T3 –
T4 Velocity™

– SAGB Gastric Band

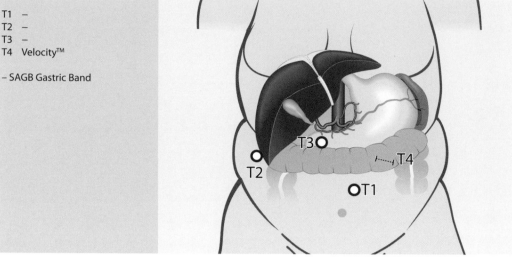

To secure the port to the fascia, depress the safety release trigger and fully compress the firing lever with the palm of the hand. With the firing lever fully compressed, release the safety release trigger. The firing lever should be locked in the fired position as shown by the lock indicator on the firing lever. Take care that the firing lever is in the locked position before lifting the applier away from the port and the incision.

> **Ensure that the firing lever is in the locked position before lifting the applier away from the port and the incision!**

Pay attention not to depress the safety release trigger once the firing lever is in the fully locked position in order not to retract the fastening hooks again. In this case the port will not release properly from the applier.

> **Note that depressing the safety release trigger once the firing lever is in the fully locked position will retract the fastening hooks and the port will not release properly from the applier!**

> **If the safety release trigger has been depressed accidentally repeat the last step to secure the port again before removing the applier!**

Remove the applier from the port and the incision. The port is left attached to the fascia; usually no securing sutures are necessary.

> **Note that it may be necessary to reposition the port during the primary SAGB Gastric Band implant procedure or during a revision procedure (→ p. 76, band erosion; p. 77, leakage from the band system; port complications)!**

> **Alternative: If appropriate fixation of the port cannot be accomplished by the integrated fastening hooks, or if an additional fixation is desired, the port can be secured in place with sutures using the three holes visible through the actuator ring in the port.**

> **Alternative: Instead of the Velocity™ Injection Port and Applier another port system can be connected to adjust the gastric band. When using another type of port system read the instruction manual carefully and become familiar with the system.**

Depressing the safety release trigger

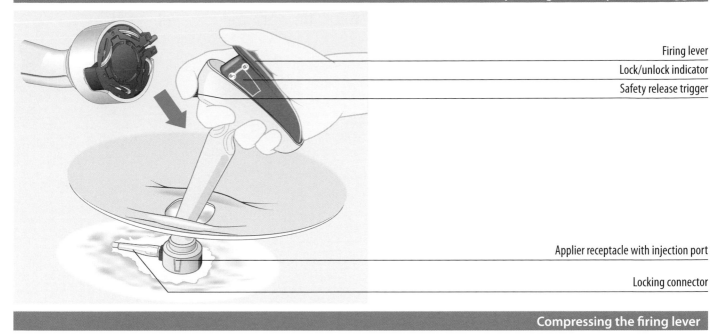

Firing lever

Lock/unlock indicator

Safety release trigger

Applier receptacle with injection port

Locking connector

Compressing the firing lever

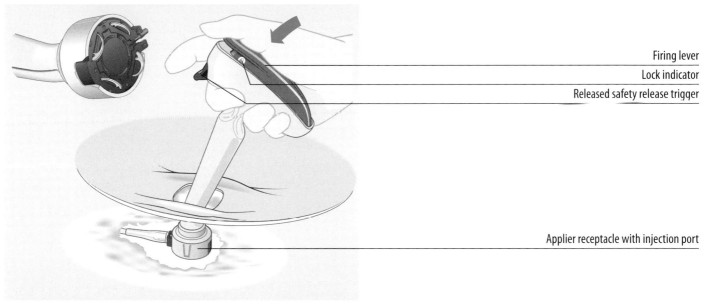

Firing lever

Lock indicator

Released safety release trigger

Applier receptacle with injection port

Lifting the applier away from the port

Firing lever

Released safety release trigger

Applier receptacle

Skin incision

Injection port

Fascia

13 Finishing the operation

T1 –
T2 –
T3 –
T4 Velocity™

– Surgical forceps
– Needle holder
– Suture scissors
– 2 Langenbeck hooks
– Fascia sutures 2–0 absorbable, polyfilament
– Subcutaneous sutures 3–0 absorbable, polyfilament, if necessary
– Skin sutures 4–0 or 5–0 absorbable, monofilament
– Dressings

– SAGB Gastric Band

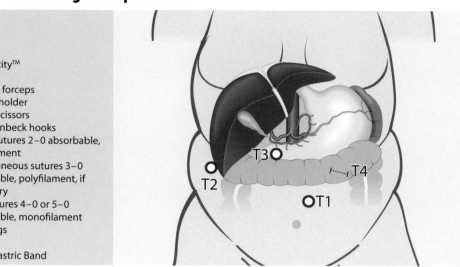

Position two Langenbeck hooks at the skin incision of T4 and re-check the correct position of the injection port and the band tubing.

Close the fascia where 10/12 mm trocars have been introduced with absorbable material in order to prevent possible hernia formation.

Then close all incisions and cover the wounds with sterile dressings following disinfection.

Alternative: Instead of skin sutures and dressings Dermabond® (Ethicon Products) can be used to close the skin incisions.

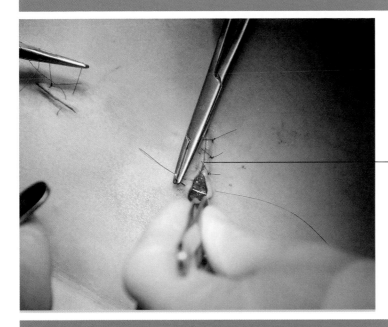

Port incision

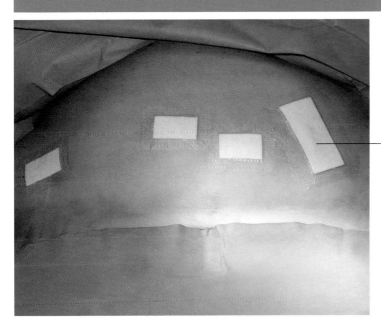

Dressings

V   MANAGEMENT OF DIFFICULT SITUATIONS AND COMPLICATIONS

In principle, the decision to proceed to laparotomy should be made too early rather than too late! In obese patients, however, the possibility of other trocar positions should be considered before converting to a conventional operation in order to gain a better view! Convert immediately if the situation cannot be controlled laparoscopically!

1   Adhesions

Separate adhesions using the HF electrode, the ultrasonic device or curved scissors as close to the abdominal wall as possible so as not to injure any organs.

2   Blood vessel injuries

a) Diffuse bleeding/bleeding from minor vessels

Coagulate the bleeding vessel with the HF electrode or the ultrasonic device. If this does not terminate the bleeding, place a clip on the bleeding vessel.

Note that if a clip has to be placed in the region of the later band position, a safe band implantation is no longer possible!

Stop any bleeding close to the gastric wall ideally with the HF electrode or the ultrasonic device or with an atraumatic transfixing suture.

b) Bleeding from major vessels

If large vessels such as the aorta, portal vein or vena cava are injured during the operation, open the abdomen immediately for vascular surgical treatment of the injury!

3   Organ injuries

In case of injuries in which the extent cannot be determined with certainty, open the abdominal cavity for open management of the injury!

a) Greater omentum

Injury to the greater omentum can occur when the Veress needle is inserted too deeply and/or without elevation of the abdominal wall. All the safety tests may be positive so that the complication can be identified only when the trocar for the scope and the scope are inserted.

Manage any bleeding that occurs with the HF electrode or the ultrasonic device. If, as a result of the insertion, the greater omentum is inflated like a tent, withdraw the trocar for the scope as far as the peritoneal margin and tap the abdomen with the flat hand. The omentum should then separate from the inside of the abdominal wall and collapse.

b) Esophagus

Injury to the esophagus is a very serious complication. Oversew the injury very carefully and then finish the operation without implanting the band. If the band has already been placed, remove it.

In case of an injury to the esophagus oversew the injury very carefully and do not implant the band!

c) Stomach

Perform gastroscopy to confirm a gastric injury and examine precisely where the lesion is located:

- If it is located in the area of the later gastric band location, oversew the defect with 2-0 absorbable material. Band implantation must not take place in this case, as band erosion can occur (→ **p. 76, band erosion**).

- If the injury to the gastric wall is outside the later band location, oversew the lesion carefully with 2-0 absorbable material and implant the band.

Suturing of the defect can be done laparoscopically or in a conventional operation, depending on the extent of the lesion.

d) Liver

Manage minor bleeding from the liver by brief compression with a swab or point contact with the HF electrode or the ultrasonic device.

In the case of major hemorrhage which can still be controlled laparoscopically, apply a hemostyptic.

e) Spleen

Bleeding from the spleen is ideally treated with the HF electrode or the ultrasonic device. Alternatively, apply a hemostyptic or perform a laparotomy, depending on the extent of the injury. Laparotomy is the exception.

f) Bowel

Bowel injuries are rare complications in gastric banding. They lead to a marked increase in the risk of infection of the band.

They are usually caused by instruments, especially by the Veress needle. Undissected adhesions can also be a cause of bowel injuries.

Manage bowel injuries by laparoscopic oversewing. If sufficient closure of the injury is not guaranteed, perform laparotomy. Irrigate the operating field gently with an antiseptic solution in order to reduce the risk of infection for the band system. As bowel resections always require a systemic antibiotic (single dose), the patient should already have antibiotic coverage (→ p. 17, I).

4   Preperitoneal air emphysema

a) Veress needle

If emphysema has occurred because of an incorrectly placed needle, remove the needle and reinsert it as described above (→ p. 28, IIc). Ensure particularly that the angle of insertion is vertical and that the abdominal wall is lifted.

b) Trocar

Withdrawing a trocar so far that its opening comes to lie in front of the peritoneum is another cause of emphysema.

In this case, under vision push the trocar back into the correct position through the existing incision.

5 Losing a swab in the abdominal cavity

After losing a swab, fix the trocar in its last position and, under vision, look for the swab where it was lost, using an atraumatic grasping forceps.

Do not change the patient's position, and do not irrigate the abdominal cavity!

If necessary, search for the swab with the C-arm or perform a laparotomy to retrieve the swab.

Do not give up searching until the swab is found!

6 Opening the omental bursa

If the omental bursa is opened, secure the correct position of the gastric band with an additional safety suture between the fundus and the pouch on the posterior wall of the stomach. Place the suture under vision as far posteriorly as possible.

Place all other safety sutures as described (→ p. 50, nodal point 9), to prevent slippage of the gastric band (→ **p. 75, pouch dilatation**).

7 Tightness of the gastric band

If the gastric band is too tight around the stomach after closing because of large quantities of perigastric fat, necrosis of the stomach wall due to excessive pressure can occur!

In this case re-open the band and close it again using the combined technique as described below.

Grasp the fatty tissue at the lesser curvature at the level of the gastric band with an atraumatic grasping forceps and separate it carefully from the gastric wall until the curvature becomes visible. Then pass the Goldfinger™ carefully through the incision at the lesser curvature side until its tip appears at the pars flaccida incision site.

Guide the Goldfinger™ with caution in order to avoid injuries to the neighboring organs and blood vessels (→ p. 65, V-2; V-3)!

Secure the suture loop of the opened gastric band in the notch of the Goldfinger™ using the atraumatic grasping forceps. Pull the Goldfinger™ with the attached band under vision slowly and carefully from the pars flaccida incision through this tunnel to the incision at the lesser curvature close to the gastric wall until the band extender flap appears at this site. If necessary, use the forceps to assist in drawing the band through.

Proceed with the closure of the band as described in nodal point 8 (p. 48).

APPENDICES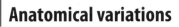

 Anatomical variations

Sample operation note

 Postoperative management

a) Analgesia
b) Mobilization
c) Nutrition
d) Discharge

 Band adjustment

a) First band adjustment
b) Further band adjustment

 Management of postoperative complications

a) Band complications
b) Port complications

Bibliography

 Keywords

 Editors

Assistants

 Titles available

Anatomical variations

Accessory hepatic artery

In about 20 % of cases an accessory hepatic artery in the region of the pars flaccida may be present. Be aware of this possible anatomical variation when making the incision in the pars flaccida.

Date:	Operating surgeon:
Patient's name:	Assistant:
Operation diagnosis: Morbid adipositas	Scrub nurse:
Operation: Laparoscopic gastric banding with the SAGB Gastric Band	Anesthetist:

Patient under general anesthesia, placed in lithotomy position with adequate padding. Skin disinfection and sterile draping, followed by a skin incision a hand's breadth below the xiphoid and 1–2 fingers paramedian on the left.

The Veress needle is inserted transmuscular through the incision and the usual safety tests are carried out. Pneumoperitoneum is then established with a pressure of 12 mmHg.

A 12-mm trocar for the scope is placed through this incision and the scope is brought into the abdomen. The patient is then placed in a reverse Trendelenburg position. A 360° view reveals no pathological changes and/or injuries. Under direct visualization a 12-mm trocar is placed in the right upper abdomen and the liver retracting device is inserted and fixed with the self-retainer. Then a 5-mm and a 15-mm trocar are placed in the right and left epigastrium, respectively, under vision.

Following a diagnostic laparoscopy the gastric calibration tube is inserted as far as the gastro-esophageal junction by the anesthetist. The pars flaccida is incised caudal to the gastro-esophageal junction and cranial to the left gastric artery. The right crus of the diaphragm is exposed and the fatty tissue medial to the right crus is then incised. The gastric calibration tube is advanced into the stomach by the anesthetist. The avascular part of the gastrophrenic ligament at the angle of His is then incised, and the left crus of the diaphragm is exposed over a distance of 1–1.5 cm.

The gastric band is carefully checked for leaks and completeness and is introduced into the abdominal cavity through the 15-mm trocar.

The retrocardial tunnel is created by gently introducing the Goldfinger™, starting from the incision at the right crus of the diaphragm retrocardially towards the incision at the angle of His. The suture loop of the gastric band is connected to the Goldfinger™. Then the gastric calibration tube is withdrawn into the esophagus by the anesthetist. Under vision, the Goldfinger™ with the attached band is carefully pulled from the angle of His through the retrocardial tunnel. The gastric band is positioned so that its balloon is oriented towards the stomach wall. The gastric band is closed.

With the first safety suture the fundus of the stomach is fixed to the left crus of the diaphragm. Two additional sutures between the fundus and the pouch are placed anteriorly. The stomach is tested for leaks, then the gastric calibration tube is removed by the anesthetist.

Following inspection of the operating field, the tubing of the gastric band is pulled out through the 15-mm trocar. The 15-mm trocar is removed under vision and the fascia at its entry site is closed. The remaining trocars are removed. The tubing of the gastric band is connected to the Velocity™ Injection Port and the port is fixed on the fascia.

Fascia and skin of the incisions are closed and the incisions are covered with sterile dressings.

Postoperative management

a) Analgesia

Take care to give adequate pain medication for fast recovery of the patient.

On day of operation give opioids as needed by the patient. From the first postoperative day prescription of simple analgesia (NSAIDs) is sufficient in most cases.

b) Mobilization

Depending on anesthetic aftereffects and circulatory stability, mobilize the patient as soon as possible postoperatively.

c) Nutrition

Day of operation: Six hours postoperatively allow the patient to drink tea in sips.

First postoperative day: After an inconspicuous X-ray control with Gastrografin, allow the patient to drink tea and eat soup and yoghurt.

Second postoperative day: For breakfast tea or coffee and crispbread with butter and jam or spread cheese is recommended. For lunch and dinner offer the patient porridge.

Third postoperative day: For breakfast tea or coffee and crispbread with butter and jam or spread cheese is recommended. Then regular diet as tolerated.

A stool softener is usually not necessary.

d) Discharge

Discharge the patient on the second or third day. Prior to discharge make sure that the patient is mobilized, has passed urine, is pain free, and is tolerating a normal diet.

Outpatient postoperative care is possible if the patient is mobilized, has passed urine, is pain free, and is tolerating fluids.

X-ray fluoroscopy device
Huber needle (20–22G, 50 mm or longer)
10-ml syringe
Water-soluble contrast agent (e.g. Iopamidol 41 %) or 0.9 % saline solution
Barium-containing contrast agent

a) First band adjustment

Perform the first band adjustment of the SAGB Gastric Band 4–6 weeks postoperatively.

Fill the band no earlier than 4–6 weeks after the operation as earlier fillings would increase the risk of slippage of the gastric band and the risk of esophageal dilatation!

Before filling the band for the first time with 3–4 ml, ensure that

- the patient needs a band filling (Some patients are fine without filling of the band. Important is the feeling of satiety and not the volume the band is filled with),

- no intestinal obstruction exists and

- no abdominal pain occurs in association with eating.

For band adjustment, position the patient in supine position on the X-ray table and disinfect the skin over the port carefully. Then bring the table into a 30°–45° reverse Trendelenburg position.

Fill the syringe with 3–4 ml of water-soluble contrast agent (e.g. Iopamidol 41 %) or sterile 0.9 % saline solution. Locate the port by palpation. Fix the port with two fingers and insert the Huber needle vertical to the skin surface into the chamber between your fingers.

Always use atraumatic Huber needles for penetration of the port septum so as not to damage the silicone membrane of the injection port!

If the injection port cannot be located in this manner, repeat the puncture under fluoroscopic control.

Aspirate the enclosed air from the band. Ensure that all air is removed from the band system before it is filled for the first time. Then inject 3–4 ml of the water-soluble contrast agent or the saline solution into the port.

Have the patient swallow barium-containing contrast agent under fluoroscopic control. Check the correct position and filling of the band:

- the angle of the band to the transverse plane should be 40°–45° and

- the contrast agent should have moved from the pouch into the stomach in a continuous flow in 1–2 peristaltic waves.

If necessary, aspirate or inject some of the water-soluble contrast agent until optimal filling can be demonstrated on the barium swallow.

Do not exceed the maximum volume of 4 ml for the first filling as this would increase the distension or dilatation risk of the esophagus!

b) Further band adjustment

Fill the gastric band step by step in order to avoid complications. The period between two fillings should be at least 3 months.

For the second and third band adjustments, first empty the band completely.
Compare the aspirated volume with the volume of fluid injected at the last filling and increase or reduce the previous filling volume according to the following plan:

+ 0.5–1 ml	In case of a weight loss of 0.5–1 kg per week and no symptoms such as obstruction or abdominal pain in association with eating.
The same volume	In case of a weight loss of more than 1 kg per week.
– 0.5–1 ml	In case of a weight loss of more than 1 kg per week and persistent obstructive symptoms such as protracted vomiting, regurgitation or inability to eat.

Take care never to fill the gastric band with a total volume of more than 9 ml, as this would increase the risk of obstruction and slippage of the gastric band!

After each further filling of the band, check immediately whether the patient can swallow. For this, have the patient drink water in small sips.

Before discharging the patient, ensure that there are no clinical signs of obstruction such as vomiting. Tell the patient to return to the clinic immediately if there are signs of obstruction, which may occur as late as 24 hours after band adjustment.

If the slightest suspicion of obstruction exists, perform a barium swallow to obtain objective evidence, as the patient's own subjective reports are often difficult to assess!

In complication-free patients with adequate weight loss, perform an annual radiological check of the band system with contrast agent.

Management of postoperative complications

a) Band complications

In case of band complications which cannot be treated directly, give the patient a lipase inhibitor to avoid weight gain until the defective band system is corrected or exchanged.

1. Pouch dilatation

- **Without slippage of the gastric band**

  Causes of this complication can be:
  - the pouch size selected during the operation is too big (> 15 ml),
  - the patient is eating too fast,
  - the patient is eating beyond a sensation of satiety,
  - the patient consumes carbonic acid-containing drinks or
  - the patient vomits violently.

  To confirm the diagnosis of an early (less than one year) pouch dilatation give a contrast agent under X-ray control.

  Treat the pouch dilatation by removing the liquid from the band's tubing system to expand the stoma. In a few cases it is possible to reverse the dilatation this way.

  If this is not successful, perform a laparoscopy and place the band again or remove it and convert to a Roux-en-Y gastric bypass.

  Unrecognized early pouch dilatation could lead to stasis esophagitis and/or weight gain.

- **With slippage of the gastric band**

  With a band slippage, a part of the distal stomach slides proximally through the band and causes occlusion or pouch dilatation.

  Causes of this complication can be:
  - placing the band inside the omental bursa without a posterior suture to the posterior wall of the stomach,
  - placing the band outside the gastrophrenic ligament,
  - incorrectly placed safety sutures or ruptured sutures due to violent vomiting.

  To confirm the diagnosis of slippage or pouch dilatation give a contrast agent under X-ray control.

  Treat the pouch dilatation or slippage by removing the liquid from the band's tubing system to expand the stoma. In a few cases it is possible to reverse the dilatation this way.

  If this is not successful, perform a laparoscopy and place the band again or exchange it.

Note that with slippage the gastric wall can become inflamed and can thus be very vulnerable!

2. Pouch rupture

Tearing of the pouch can occur in case of a pre-existing pouch dilatation, sliding of the stomach wall with strangulation and necrosis, or excessive consumption of carbonic acid-containing drinks.

Manage this injury by oversewing the defect laparoscopically with absorbable material. If necessary excise the defect, suture it, and place a drainage in the left subphrenium.

3. Stoma occlusion

In stoma occlusion an obstruction within the opening of the gastric band exists due to inadequately chewed food.

In this case, remove the filling liquid from the band and then have the patient drink under X-ray control. If this eliminates the occlusion, refill the band.

If this is not successful, perform a laparoscopy and remove the band.

If the occlusion lasts for more than six hours, refill the band only after a few days because of the pouch dilatation and the possible inflammatory component.

4. Band erosion

Band erosion is the term given to migration of the band into the stomach.

> **Note that band erosion is the postoperative complication with the most serious consequences!**

Possible causes are:
- primary intraoperative injury to the wall of the stomach,

- pressure necrosis as a result of excessive filling of the band, or

- secondary infection of the band system.

Confirm the diagnosis by gastroscopy.

Remove the band either gastroscopically or laparoscopically, or remove only the port.

- For gastroscopic gastric band removal:
  When at least one third of the band has migrated into the stomach remove the band by gastroscopy. To do so first disconnect the tubing system from the port. Then divide and remove the band. Perform a check for leaks in the gastric wall with Gastrografin.

  If the gastric wall has been injured, perform a laparoscopy and suture the defect with absorbable material. Place a drainage in the left subphrenium.

  Finally, remove the port (→ p. 77, port rotation).

- For laparoscopic gastric band removal:
  Remove the gastric band laparoscopically if there are complications such as hemorrhage, reflux or dysphagia. To do so first disconnect the tubing system from the port. Perform a gastrotomy, then divide and remove the gastric band laparoscopically. Close the stomach in a single layer with absorbable suture material and check for leaks by gastroscopy or air insufflation. Finally, remove the port (→ p. 77, port rotation).

- For port removal only:
  If the patient is asymptomatic with complete band erosion, simply disconnect and remove the port (→ p. 77, port rotation). The band will then be excreted naturally.

> **Consider an excretion of the gastric band naturally only if the particularly softly structured Swedish Adjustable Gastric Band (SAGB) was used!**

5. Band infection

An infection can arise primarily by contamination of the band during implantation and secondarily from port infection or inoculation of bacteria if the safety sutures pass transmurally.

In case of band infection, remove the entire band system immediately under systemic antibiotic coverage. Implantation of a new band is possible after a few weeks.

6. Leakage from the band system

A leak in the band system usually becomes evident by an asymptomatic weight gain.

In order to examine the port and tubing system for major leaks, inject a defined volume of liquid (at least 5 ml) and try to re-aspirate it completely. If this test is negative, inject a contrast agent (e.g. Iopamiro) to detect smaller leaks. The smallest leaks can be detected by a thallium-201 isotope scan.

In case of a leak of the port, remove the port under local anesthesia (→ p. 77, port rotation).

If the leak is located anywhere in the inflatable part of the band, remove the entire system.

If the leakage is located in the tubing system close to the port, remove the damaged section of the tube and reposition the port if necessary.

b) Port complications

1. Port infection

Perform gastroscopy with every port infection, as the infection can be due to band erosion.

- **With band erosion**

  Remove the port (→ p. 77, port rotation) and disinfect the infected area carefully with a mounted swab. Remove the gastric band as described above (→ p. 76, band erosion). Ensure an adequate systemic antibiotic coverage.

- **Without band erosion**

  Remove the port (→ p. 77, port rotation) and fill the gastric band with the last filling volume applied. Disinfect the infected area carefully with a mounted swab. Then shorten and close the tubing system and submerge it into the abdominal cavity. Ensure an adequate systemic antibiotic coverage.

  Perform a laparoscopy after about 8–12 months to implant a new port at another trocar port site.

2. Port penetration

Reposition the port (→ p. 77, port rotation) operatively before damage to the epidermis occurs.

Note that this complication is avoidable if the port is consistently placed on the fascia!

3. Port rotation

- **Port**

  Replace an old port with a Velocity™ Injection Port as described in nodal point 12 (p. 56).

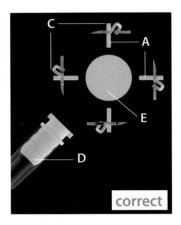

correct

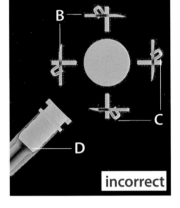

incorrect

- **Velocity™ Injection Port**

If port rotation is suspected, obtain an X-ray image of the port.

The port has five radiopaque parts which can be used to determine the port orientation:
A: Alignment pin
B: Fastening hook
C: Link
D: Locking connector
E: Reservoir base

The correct orientation of the port shows the location of the link to the right of the alignment pin if the alignment pin is envisioned in the 12 o'clock position.

If the port is in an incorrect orientation, the link is on the left of the alignment pin when the pin is envisioned in the 12 o'clock position, and the port is inverted upside down.

Incorrect orientation may necessitate repositioning of the port with additional surgery.

To reposition or remove the Velocity™ Injection Port, clear tissue growth around the port and the fastening hooks, then remove the port as desribed below.

Place the applier receptacle over the port. Make sure that the gray firing lever of the applier is fully compressed and locked in the fired position as shown by the lock indicator on the firing lever and that the guide notch aligns with the connection housing.

Apply slight downward pressure to the applier and depress the safety release trigger in order to retract the fastening hooks. The firing lever automatically snaps to a partially open position.

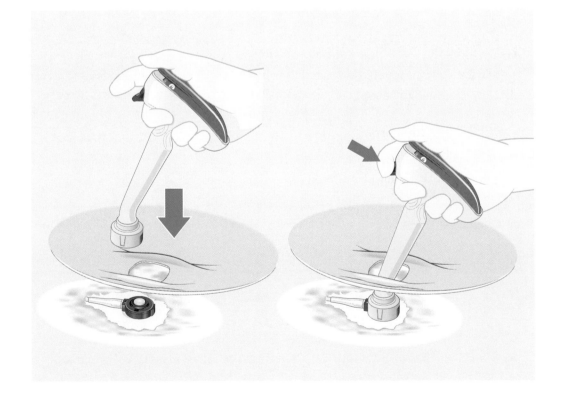

Continue to maintain slight downward pressure to the applier with one hand while pulling the firing lever upwards with the other hand until it is in the fully unlocked position as indicated on the firing lever. The safety release trigger will lock the firing lever in this position.

If the port has to be removed from the incision, remove the applier at an angle such that the tubing and the locking connector do not touch tissue, in order not to pull out the port of the applier receptacle.

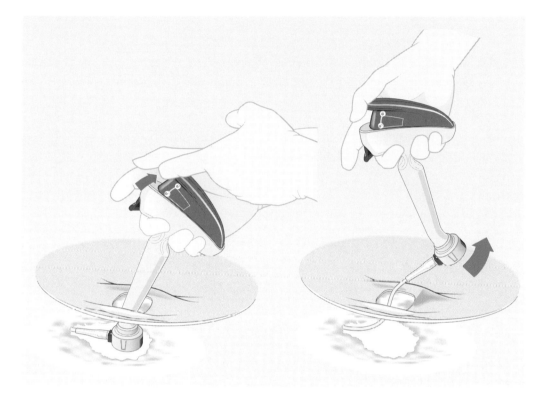

After cleaning the freed port, reposition it on the fascia and attach it again as described in nodal point 12 (p. 56). Alternatively, implant a new Velocity™ Injection Port.

4. Disconnection of the port and tubing system

To check the port and the tubing system for leaks, inject a defined volume of liquid (at least 5 ml) and try to re-aspirate it completely.

Expose the port under local anesthesia and reconnect the tube to the chamber. If necessary, secure the locking connector by tying non-absorbable suture material around it tightly.

Bibliography

Abu-Abeid S. & Szold A. (1999). Results and complications of laparoscopic adjustable gastric banding: an early and intermediate experience. *Obesity Surgery*, 9: 188.

Arora S., Aggarwal R., Sevdalis N., Moran A., Sirimanna P., Kneebone R. & Darzi A. (2010). Development and validation of mental practice as a training strategy for laparoscopic surgery. *Surgical Endoscopy*, 24: 179–187.

Belachew M., Jacquet P., Lardinois F. & Karler C. (1993). Vertical banded gastroplasty vs adjustable silicone gastric banding in the treatment of morbid obesity: a preliminary report. *Obesity Surgery*, 3: 275–278.

Benninghoff A. & Drenkhahn D. (2008). *Anatomie. Makroskopische Anatomie, Histologie, Embryologie, Zellbiologie, Band 1*. München: Elsevier.

Berrevoet F., Pattyn P., Cardon A., de Ryck F., Hesse U.J. & de Hemptinne B. (1998). Retrospective analysis of laparoscopic gastric banding technique: short-term and mid-term follow-up. *Obesity Surgery*, 9: 272–275.

Carpenter W.B. (1874). *Principles of Mental Physiology: With their Applications to the Training and Discipline of the Mind and the Study of its Comorbid Conditions*. London: Henry S. King & Co.

Ceelen W., Walder J., Cardon A., Van Renterghem K., Hesse U., El Malt M. & Pattyn P. (2003). Surgical treatment of severe obesity with a low-pressure adjustable gastric band: experimental data and clinical results in 625 patients. *Annals of Surgery*, 237: 10–16.

Chelala E., Cadière G.B., Favretti F., Himpens J., Vertruyen M., Bruyns J., Maroquin L. & Lise M. (1997). Conversions and complications in 185 laparoscopic adjustable silicone gastric banding cases. *Surgical Endoscopy*, 11: 268–271.

Elmore U., Restuccia A., Perrotta N., Polito D., De Leo A., Silecchia G. & Basso N. (1998). Laparoscopic adjustable silicone gastric banding (LASGB): analyses of 64 consecutive patients. *Obesity Surgery*, 8: 399.

Feltz D.L. & Landers D.M. (1983). The effects of mental practice on motor skill learning and performance: a meta-analysis. *Journal of Sport Psychology*, 5: 25–57.

Forsell P. & Hellers G. (1997). The Swedish adjustable gastric banding for morbid obesity – nine-year experience and a four-year follow-up of patients operated with a new adjustable band. *Obesity Surgery*, 7: 345–351.

Fried M., Miller K. & Kormanova K. (2004). Literature review of comparative studies of complications with Swedish Band and Lap-Band®. *Obesity Surgery*, 14: 256–260.

Güler A.K., Immenroth M., Berg T., Bürger T. & Gawad K.A. (2006). Evaluation einer neu konzipierten Operationsfibel durch den Vergleich mit einer klassischen chirurgischen Operationslehre. *Posterpräsentation auf dem 123. Kongress der Deutschen Gesellschaft für Chirurgie vom 02.–05. Mai 2006 in Berlin*.

Hell E. & Miller K. (1999). Laparoscopic treatment of complications after adjustable gastric banding. *Obesity Surgery*, 9: 352–353.

Hell E. & Miller K. (2000). *Morbide Adipositas. Klinik und chirurgische Therapie.* Landsberg: Ecomed Verlag.

Hell E., Miller K., Moorehead M.K. & Samuels N. (2000). Comparison of standard Roux-en-Y gastric bypass, vertical banded gastroplasty and laparoscopic adjustable silicone gastric banding. *Obesity Surgery*, 10: 214–219.

Hell E. & Miller K. (2002). Development, state of the art and future perspectives of surgery for morbid obesity. *Zentralblatt für Chirurgie*, 127: 1025–1031.

Hell E. & Miller K. (2002). Adipositaschirurgie im interdisziplinären und rechtlichen Spannungsfeld. *Zentralblatt für Chirurgie*, 127: 1032–1034.

Hell E. & Miller K. (2002). Criteria for selection of patients for bariatric surgery. *Zentralblatt für Chirurgie*, 127: 1035–1037.

Immenroth M. (2003). *Mentales Training in der Medizin. Anwendung in der Chirurgie und Zahnmedizin.* Hamburg: Kovac.

Immenroth M., Bürger T., Brenner J., Kemmler R., Nagelschmidt R., Eberspächer H. & Troidl H. (2005). Mentales Training in der Chirurgie. *Der Chirurg* BDC, 44: 21–25.

Immenroth M., Bürger T., Brenner J., Nagelschmidt R., Eberspächer H. & Troidl H. (2007). Mental Training in surgical education: a randomized controlled trial. *Annals of Surgery*, 245: 385–391.

Immenroth M., Eberspächer H., Nagelschmidt M., Troidl H., Bürger T., Brenner J., Berg T., Müller M. & Kemmler R. (2005). Mentales Training in der Chirurgie – Sicherheit durch ein besseres Training. Design und erste Ergebnisse einer Studie. *MIC*, 14: 69–74.

Immenroth M., Eberspächer H. & Hermann H.D. (2008). Training kognitiver Fertigkeiten. In J. Beckmann & M. Kellmann (Hrsg.), *Enzyklopädie der Psychologie (D, V, 2). Anwendungen der Sportpsychologie* (119–176). Göttingen: Hogrefe.

Jung G. (1996). *Pflegestandards in der minimal-invasiven Chirurgie.* Hannover: Schlütersche Verlagsgesellschaft.

Klaiber C., Metzger A. & Forsell P. (2000). Laparoskopisches gastric banding. *Chirurg*, 71: 146–151.

Köckerling F. (1995). Offene Laparoskopie. In K. Kremer, W. Platzer & H.W. Schreiber (Hrsg.), *Chirurgische Operationslehre. Minimal-invasive Chirurgie, Band 7, Teil 2* (54–58). Stuttgart, New York: Georg Thieme Verlag.

Kunath U. & Memari B. (1995). Laparoskopisches "Gastric Banding" zur Behandlung der pathologischen Adipositas. *Chirurg*, 66: 1263–1267.

Leonhardt H. (1987) Innere Organe. In H. Leonhardt, B. Tillmann, G. Töndury & K. Zilles (Hrsg.), *Anatomie des Menschen, Band 2.* Stuttgart, New York: Georg Thieme Verlag.

Lotze R.H. (1852). *Medicinische Psychologie und Physiologie der Seele.* Leipzig: Weidmann'sche Buchhandlung.

Mazarguil P., Bertrand J.C. & Peraldi D. (1997). Laparoscopic adjustable silicone gastric banding (LASGB) for the treatment of morbid obesity. *Obesity Surgery,* 7: 299.

Miller G.A. (1956). The magical number seven plus or minus two: some limits on our capacity for processing information. *Psychological Review,* 63: 81–97.

Miller K. (2002). Adipositaschirurgie. *Chirurgie,* 1: 10–18.

Miller K. (2003). Laparoskopische Operationsverfahren bei morbider Adipositas. *Journal für Ernährungsmedizin,* 5: 5–11.

Miller K. (2004). Obesity: surgical options. Best Practice & Research. *Clinical Gastroenterology,* 18: 1147–1165.

Miller K. (2005). Laparoscopic bariatric surgery in the treatment of morbid obesity. *Endoscopic Review,* 10: 73–82.

Miller K. (2008). Evolution of gastric band implantation and port fixation techniques. *Surgery for Obesity and Related Diseases,* 4: S22–S30.

Miller K. & Hell E. (1999). Laparoscopic adjustable gastric banding. *Acta Chirurgica Austriaca,* 31: 152–155.

Miller K. & Hell E. (1999). Laparoscopic adjustable gastric banding: a prospective four-year follow-up study. *Obesity Surgery,* 9: 183–187.

Miller K. & Pump A. (2008). Mechanical versus suture fixation of the port in adjustable gastric banding procedures: a prospective randomized blinded study. *Surgical Endoscopy,* 22: 2478–2484.

Miller K., Pump A. & Hell E. (2007). Vertical banded gastroplasty versus adjustable gastric banding: prospective long-term follow-up study. *Surgery for Obesity and Related Diseases,* 3: 84–90.

Miller K., Rettenbacher L. & Hell E. (1996). Adjustments and leak detection of the adjustable silicone gastric band (ASGB) and Lap-Band® adjustable gastric band system. *Obesity Surgery,* 6: 406–411.

Mittermair R.P., Weiss H., Nehoda H., Kirchmayr W. & Aigner F. (2003). Laparoscopic Swedish adjustable gastric banding: six-year follow-up and comparison to other laparoscopic bariatric procedures. *Obesity Surgery,* 13: 412–417.

Netter F.H. (2003). *Atlas of Human Anatomy.* Teterboro, New Jersey: Icon Learning Systems.

Steffen R., Biertho L., Ricklin T., Piec G. & Horber F.F. (2003). Laparoscopic Swedish adjustable banding: a five-year prospective study. *Obesity Surgery,* 13: 404–411.

Weiner R. (1999). *Manual Laparoskopisches Gastric Banding. Die Behandlung der morbiden Adipositas.* Heidelberg, Leipzig: Johann Ambrosius Barth Verlag.

Weiss H., Nehoda H., Labeck B., Peer R. & Aigner F. (2000). Gastroscopic band removal after intragastral migration of adjustable gastric band: a new minimal invasive technique. *Obesity Surgery,* 10: 167–170.

Marc Immenroth, PhD

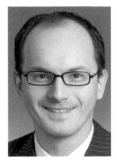

- Studied Psychology (Diploma) and Sports Science (Master) in Heidelberg, Germany
- 1999–2006 Sports Psychologist (including consultant to many German top athletes during their preparation for the World Championships and Olympics) and Industrial Psychologist (including consultant to Lufthansa Inc.)
- 2000 Research Scientist at the University of Greifswald, Germany (Polyclinic for Restorative Dentistry and Periodontology)
- 2001–2004 Research Scientist at the University of Heidelberg, Germany (Institute of Sports and Sports Science)
- 2002 Doctorate in Psychology at the University of Heidelberg, Germany
- 2005–2006 Assistant Lecturer at the University of Giessen, Germany (Institute of Sports)
- 2006–2008 Assistant Professor at the University of Greifswald, Germany (Institute of Sports)
- 2006–2009 European Clinical Studies Manager at Ethicon Endo-Surgery (Europe) GmbH in Norderstedt, Germany
- 2009–2010 Marketing Manager and Sales Support at Ethicon Products, Johnson & Johnson MEDICAL GmbH in Norderstedt, Germany
- Since 2010 Senior Marketing Manager EP Austria & Plus Platform & Synthetic Absorbables D-A-CH, Johnson & Johnson MEDICAL GmbH in Norderstedt, Germany

Focus of Research and Work
- Mental Training in Sport, Surgery and Aviation
- Virtual Reality in Surgical Education
- Coping with Emotion and Stress

Author of many scientific articles and textbooks in psychology, sports science and medicine

Jürgen Brenner, M.D.

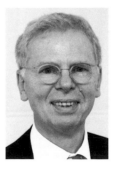

- Studied Medicine in Hamburg, Germany
- 1972 Doctorate in Medicine at the University of Hamburg, Germany
- 1972 Institute for Neuroanatomy, University of Hamburg, Germany
- 1974 Senior Resident at the Department of Surgery of the General Hospital Hamburg-Wandsbek, Germany
- 1981 Medical Director of the Department for Colorectal and Trauma Surgery at St. Adolf Stift Hospital in Reinbek, Germany
- 1987 Director for Surgical Research of Ethicon Inc. in Norderstedt, Germany
- 1989 Director of European Surgical Institute and Vice President Professional Education Europe of Ethicon Endo-Surgery (Europe) GmbH in Norderstedt, Germany
- 2004 Managing Director at Ethicon Endo-Surgery Germany in Norderstedt, Germany
- Since 2008 Director of European Surgical Institute in Norderstedt, Germany

Assistants

Dr. Carl GmbH

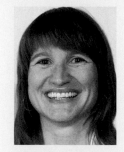

Birgit Wahl, M.D.
Medical Writer

European Surgical Institute (ESI)

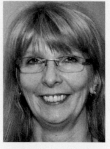

Maike Aukstinnis
Course Coordinator
Medical Education

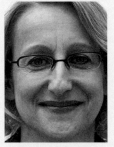

Astrid Künemund
Manager Course &
Congress Organization
CME Courses

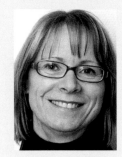

Annegret Röhling
Assistant ESI Director

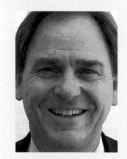

Detlev Ruge, Manager
Audio & Visual Technologies

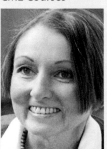

Sabine Schroeder
Course & Congress Organization
CME Courses/CME
Medical Content

**Ethicon Endo-Surgery
Johnson & Johnson
MEDICAL GmbH**

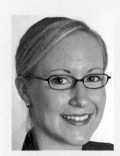

Ann-Katrin Güler, M.D.
Consultant Medical Products

Titles available

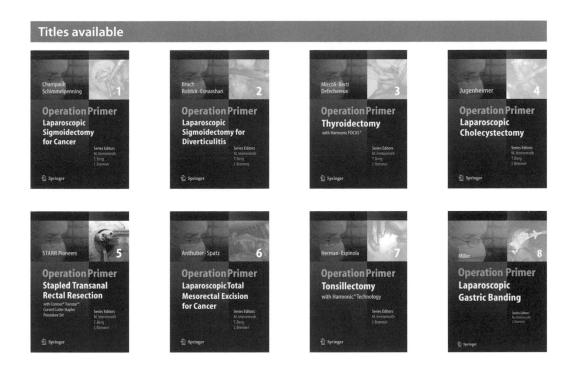

Volume 1: Laparoscopic Sigmoidectomy for Cancer   ISBN 978-3-540-78453-1

Volume 2: Laparoscopic Sigmoidectomy for Diverticulitis   ISBN 978-3-540-78451-7

Volume 3: Thyroidectomy with Harmonic FOCUS®   ISBN 978-3-540-85163-9

Volume 4: Laparoscopic Cholecystectomy   ISBN 978-3-540-92961-1

Volume 5: Stapled Transanal Rectal Resection with
       Contour® Transtar™ Curved Cutter Stapler Procedure Set   ISBN 978-3-540-92958-1

Volume 6: Laparoscopic Total Mesorectal Excision for Cancer   ISBN 978-3-642-04730-5

Volume 7: Tonsillectomy with Harmonic® Technology   ISBN 978-3-642-12747-2

Volume 8: Laparoscopic Gastric Banding   ISBN 978-3-642-19274-6

Titles in preparation

Open Total Mesorectal Excision for Rectal Cancer

Laparoscopic Gastric Bypass Procedure

Laparoscopic Gastric Sleeve Procedure

VATS-Lobectomy

Laparoscopic Hysterectomy

NOTES

NOTES

NOTES

NOTES